❧ Praise for ❧
The Perfect Metabolism Plan

"*The Perfect Metabolism Plan* busts powerful, long-standing myths that have stood in the way of achieving good health and balanced weight for decades. This book gives the reader a true understanding of how food affects them and why not all calories are created equal. An approachable, fun, and empowering action plan that teaches you how to eat real food and regain your health and metabolism for the long-term!"

—CHRISTA ORECCHIO, CHN author of *180 Ways to Use Food as Medicine* and *How to Conceive Naturally*

"Important, accessible, smart. This book offer a realistic plan that gently coaches the reader while exposing the underlying causes of weight problems and virtually every disease. This is the book every doctor should give their patient, and anyone interested in health should have on the shelf. Brava!"

—PETER BONGIORNO, ND, LAc, author of *How Come They're Happy and I'm Not?*

"The Perfect Metabolism Plan brings simplicity to complexity and applied science to your life to master your health. Sara has the background, training, and credentials to teach us how to make your metabolism and well-being the perfect 10. This book stands out among similar books for its readability, accuracy, and practicality."

—MARK HOUSTON MD, MS, MSc, associate clinical professor of medicine, Vanderbilt University School of Medicine, author of *What Your Doctor May Not Tell You About Heart Disease*

"Sara Vance has written an intriguing book that creatively examines modern ideas about health and wellness and the various facets influencing metabolism. Her stance on choosing whole foods over processed foods, developing a non-inflammatory diet, and learning to exercise smarter should be embraced by anyone looking to make lasting lifestyle changes."

—JULIA B. GREER, MD, MPH, assistant professor of medicine, University of Pittsburgh School of Medicine, co-director of the medical school course Digestion and Nutrition, author of *The Anti-Cancer Cookbook* and *The Anti-Breast Cancer Cookbook*

The
Perfect
Metabolism
Plan

The Perfect Metabolism Plan

Restore Your Energy and Reach Your Ideal Weight

Sara Vance

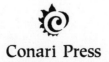

Conari Press

This edition first published in 2015 by Conari Press
Red Wheel/Weiser, LLC
With offices at:
665 Third Street, Suite 400
San Francisco, CA 94107
www.redwheelweiser.com

ISBN: 978-1-57324-643-9

Library of Congress Cataloging-in-Publication Data
Vance, Sara.
The perfect metabolism plan : the 10 keys to unlock your ideal weight and virant health without dieting/Sara Vance.
    pages cm
Summary: "Vance offers 10 proven keys for fixing or resetting your metabolism: 1. Break Up with Sugar 2. Fix Your Fats (eat healthy fats) 3. Heal Your Gut (probiotics) 4. Identify Food Intolerances (foods that make you foggy, fatigued, sick, and fat) 5. Lose the Toxins (in household products, body care products, etc.) 6. Put Out the Fire (beware acidic foods and other foods that cause inflammation) 7. Stop the Madness (stress) 8. Ditch the Convenience Foods (even the so-called healthy ones) 9. Hydrate! 10. Exercise Smarter (Not Harder)"—Provided by publisher.
  ISBN 978-1-57324-643-9 (paperback)
  1. Weight loss. 2. Metabolism. 3. Health. I. Title.
  RM222.2.V335 2015
  613.2'5—dc23
                              2014041756

Cover design by Jim Warner
Author photograph of author © Amy Casson Photography
Interior by Maureen Forys, Happenstance Type-O-Rama
Typeset in Warnock Pro and Optima

Printed in the United States of America
EBM
10 9 8 7 6 5 4 3 2 1

❧ Dedication ❧

This book is dedicated to my dad, Dr. Robert Corry. He was an organ transplant surgeon, a pioneer in the combination kidney/pancreas transplant, and a great father. I was always so proud to say that he was a doctor—he literally was saving lives! My dad's patients were very sick, because in order to qualify for a transplant, their condition had to be very advanced. He saw firsthand the terrible toll that advanced diabetes and other diseases take on the human body—including kidney failure. Those who received a new organ got a new lease on life. My dad was passionate about his work and his patients, and he always brought his unique sense of humor along with him as he made rounds at the hospital.

I sometimes think about how he'd probably get a chuckle out of the fact that his daughter, who was overweight as a child, loved sugar and hot dogs, avoided most vegetables, and even refused to try a shrimp for $20 once, was now teaching people how to cut out the sugar, eat lots of veggies, and fix their metabolism!

I wish he were alive today because I think he'd be interested in discussing nutritional approaches to health and disease prevention.

This book is for you, Dad.

I too have found my passion for helping people get a new lease on life—through nutrition!

❧ Contents ❧

❧ Acknowledgments ❧

No Army can stop an idea whose time has come.

—VICTOR HUGO

When I started, I had no idea what a massive task it is to write a book! I just want to take a moment to say thank you to the following people, without whom this book would not have been written:

Thank you so much to my husband and family, who certainly have listened to more than their fair share of information about nutrition and served as guinea pigs and taste-testers for many recipes. My husband Jeff has supported me through it all, taking the kids on adventures so I could stay home and write, and looking the other way when the laundry was piling up (or folding it). But above all, he encouraged me, believed in me, and supported me.

Thank you to my sister and business partner for being there for me all along the way. She has believed in me (even during the times when I didn't) and reached out to her network of connections who have been instrumental in this book coming into being. Cath, you are awesome and inspiring!

A big thanks to Patricia Karpas, who believed in me and my vision and introduced me to Red Wheel/Weiser and Conari Press. Just as my proposal was being accepted, she shared the above quote with me from Victor Hugo. Patricia has always amazed me with her wonderful spirit, spark, and ability to execute.

Thank you to everyone at Red Wheel, especially Caroline Pincus, my editor-extraordinaire at Red Wheel for taking a chance on me, a first-time author, and for making this book more accessible, readable, and understandable.

To my mom, who showed me that it is possible to have a career and be a good mom. She always has an open mind, is interested in natural approaches to health, and sees the glass as half full.

To my dear friend Hillary Patton for keeping me grounded and all your support.

To Jenny Gilcrest, my friend and PR manager. You are super creative and have the biggest heart—your support and friendship through all these years means the world to me.

To Tiffany at *San Diego Living*, for giving me my first opportunity to share my tips on TV!

To everyone at Fox 5 San Diego and Leslie Marcus, for having me on the Fox 5 show for the past 4 years to share my knowledge and information with San Diegans.

To my sister-in-law Julie, an amazing nutritionist and yoga teacher, for giving me the idea to start up my own group cleanse and helping me get going. I don't know if I would have created my program without your encouragement and support!

To my friends, clients, and everyone who has participated in my Perfect Metabolism programs, to those who have recommended it to others over the years, and to those who are just beginning to embark on their program. *You* are the reason I created this program! Helping others improve their health is the biggest reward. Thank you for trusting in me and Perfect Metabolism.

⚜ An Important Note ⚜

The information contained in this book should not be construed as medical advice nor is it intended to diagnose or treat symptoms, diseases, or individuals. If you have a known or suspected health condition or are under a doctor's care, please consult with a qualified health care professional before beginning this program or implementing any of the suggestions. If you are taking prescription medication or have an existing condition, please check with your doctor/pharmacist before taking any of the mentioned herbs, teas, or supplements to ensure there are no possible interactions or contraindications. Persons taking prescription medications should not stop without consulting with their doctor. The information in this book is presented to help guide you to your ideal health and serve as a supplement to, not a replacement for, medical advice. *The Perfect Metabolism Plan* readers assume all risks, whether or not such risks were created or exacerbated by the information contained in this book. This program is not designed for children, pregnant or lactating women, or persons with serious medical conditions.

And finally, great care has been taken to provide accurate and sound information. If any errors are found, please contact *info@perfect metabolism.com*. For additional resources and recipes, visit *www.perfect metabolism.com*. Any supplemental information or corrections will also be posted there.

❧ Introduction ❧
Why Diets Don't Work

Do you ever find yourself wondering why some people can eat anything they want and not gain weight? While others practically just sniff a piece of cake and gain a pound? Or why, despite strict dieting or intense exercising, you just can't seem to drop the extra weight stuck right in your midsection? Or maybe you are able to lose weight but wonder why you just can't seem to keep it off for long.

It all comes down to the metabolism.

How optimized our metabolism is affects pretty much everything: our cellular functions, hunger, hormones, detoxification channels, energy, risk of disease, the pace at which we physically age, and of course, our weight. The person who can "have her cake and eat it too" just has a more optimized metabolism. A woman who looks younger than someone else the same age likely has a more balanced metabolism. The person who is working out in the gym but can't lose any weight is experiencing the effects of a metabolism that is "out of sync."

Many people blame themselves or a lack of willpower for not being able to lose or keep weight off. But what they don't know is . . .

They didn't fail, their diet did.

Why Diets Don't Work

We count calories, cut fat, eat everything in moderation, try to exercise more and eat less—because we have been told that is what we need to do to lose weight. But many of these common approaches don't work, or worse, they can backfire—increasing hunger, slowing down our metabolism, elevating blood sugar, and negatively impacting our hormones. Even though dieting and calorie restriction might be effective for some people in the short run, unless the metabolism is reset, any weight loss will be fleeting. Let's take a look at some of the most common reasons diets fail.

Eight Common Weight Loss Myths/Mistakes

Myth 1: "We need to take in fewer calories than we burn each day."

It makes sense mathematically: bring in fewer calories than you expend in order to lose weight. Calorie-counting would work great if our bodies were calculators. Unfortunately, we are not that simple. First, all calories are not created equal; a fat calorie is different from a carbohydrate calorie in how it is processed in the body. Second, our hormones interact differently with different types of calories. If our hormones are not working ideally—as with conditions like insulin or leptin resistance—the body will not effectively deal with certain types of calories. So calorie counts can end up being irrelevant if the underlying metabolism is imbalanced. Also cutting calories too drastically can end up backfiring, because the metabolism slows down in response, leading to weight gain, and in some cases muscle mass loss: the opposite of what we want to achieve.

Myth 2: "Low-fat foods are better for my health and weight."

For decades we all fell for this one hook, line, and sinker! At first glimpse, it also makes sense: eating fats makes you gain weight and clogs your arteries. But the truth is, dietary fat does not make us fat or clog our arteries (well, okay—there are certain fats that do, which we need to avoid like the plague, like trans fats). In general, diets that are too low in fat make us hungrier, spike our blood sugar, and lead to nutrient deficiencies, weight gain and even dangerous conditions like insulin resistance, mood disorders, gallbladder trouble, and prediabetes. Low-fat diets can even age us prematurely! Seeing through the myth that low-fat foods are healthier is critical to gaining control over our metabolism, and because we have been brainwashed for so long, it can be one of the hardest ones to let go of. Chapter two details which fats are healthy and which ones to avoid at all costs (*they may not be the ones you think!*).

Myth 3: *"Diet drinks are good if you want to lose weight."*

I used to buy into the diet soda myth big time. There are no calories, so diet sodas won't cause weight gain, right? We want to believe we can drink or eat something sweet without impacting our weight or health, but dig a little deeper and you'll find that studies have linked artificial sweeteners to increased hunger, insulin problems, diabetes, and weight gain. Artificial sweeteners are on average approximately 200 times sweeter than sugar, which stimulates our sweet tooth and causes us to eat more, not less. It is thought that artificial sweeteners confuse our regulatory systems, so our brain does not register that it has eaten something sweet. And there are negative side effects too, according to Dr. Joseph Mercola, the FDA has received over 10,000 complaints about aspartame side effects.

Myth 4: *"Everything in moderation."*

If I only had a nickel for every time someone said this! Using this rule we could say "a moderate amount of alcohol" is okay for an alcoholic—because hey, *everything* is okay in moderation! Okay, I know I am being a little dramatic, but as you will learn in chapter one, some studies have found sugar to be as addictive as cocaine! What *"everything* in moderation" ignores is that many ingredients and chemicals in our foods are designed to be highly addictive, so we will continue to come back for more. Certain foods negatively affect our hormones, which tell the body to store them as fat. Consuming highly processed foods or foods that we are intolerant to can cause food addictions and inflammation, and can increase our risk for diseases. So for many people, there is no such thing as a "moderate" amount of sugar, wheat, or highly processed foods.

Myth 5: *"I just need to eat less and exercise more."*

This is similar to the calorie theory: if we exercise and burn more calories than we take in, we will lose weight. There *is* a little truth to this one. Exercise is very important if we want a healthy metabolism. But as you will learn in chapter ten, not all exercise is created equal. Many people think doing lots of cardio to "burn off" calories is the way to go. But too much cardio can actually backfire, causing our stress hormones to elevate, which can lead to weight gain! People also sometimes use exercise as an excuse to eat poorly; they trick themselves into thinking they can have that ice cream sundae and then hit the gym to burn it off. Trying to offset a nutrient-deficient diet with exercise will definitely backfire, and it might just lead to adrenal fatigue, osteoporosis, and accelerated aging. Learn how to exercise smarter, not harder in chapter ten.

Myth 6: "Whole wheat is healthier."

For years, the foundation of the American diet was grains; the food pyramid encouraged us to eat plenty of these each and every day. And if we wanted to be "healthy," we of course chose whole wheat, because it had the fiber and was less processed than white. But we now know that eating wheat, whole or not, can underlie a growing list of health complaints from weight gain to digestive troubles, autoimmune conditions, ADHD, infertility, heart disease, and even Alzheimer's and dementia. Wheat is not the only culprit, but it carries that cultural resistance. Without identifying and removing from our diet the foods that we are sensitive to, our weight loss success will likely be short-lived, and our list of health complaints will grow. Chapter four provides more information about food sensitivities and how they could be thwarting all our attempts to lose weight. In part two of this book, you will be guided through a food elimination diet to help you determine if intolerances could be affecting your weight and health.

Myth 7: "I am over forty, so I am just stuck with a slow metabolism."

It is a common misconception that we are stuck with our metabolism. Yes, our metabolism does generally slow down as we age, but is it not simply a by-product of getting older. The effectiveness of our metabolism has a lot to do with the culmination of the diet and lifestyle choices we have made over the decades. That is actually good news because it is possible to reboot our metabolism—even after age forty—if we have the right information. The Perfect Metabolism Plan provides ten keys to help you to unlock and reboot your metabolism.

Myth 8: "I am just weak; I don't have the motivation to stick to a diet and lose weight."

If you are working hard without results, your problem is not a lack of motivation. Your metabolic wires are crossed, in large part because of all these nutrition myths you have been following. When your metabolism is out of balance, your hunger and cravings are out of control, and your body is in sugar-burning and fat-storage mode. This makes it next to impossible to maintain a healthy weight. How can you get good results using bad information?

Too many of us have bought into these nutrition myths because we were given the wrong information about how to maintain a healthy weight and reduce the risk of disease. Once I realized that we've all been saddling ourselves with false blame, I knew I had to write this book. I want to help you—and the millions of others like you—to stop beating yourself up about your weight. I want to put an end to the wrong impression you are carrying that you are weak or unmotivated and the guilt you feel each time you succumb to your cravings. I was there myself once.

You might be scratching your head right now and wondering: if none of these things work, then what does? The issue at the core that needs fixing is the metabolism.

Creating a Perfect Metabolism

Trying to lose weight by dieting and calorie-counting is like putting a broken arm in a sling without resetting it first. That sling is a temporary Band-Aid solution to a deeper problem. Without resetting, when you take the broken arm out of the sling, it is still broken. Dieting is a temporary measure that lasts only as long as your willpower can stand. Just like the broken arm, a broken metabolism needs to be reset to achieve permanent and lasting weight loss. The real secret to maintaining a healthy weight is to get to the root of the problem—the metabolism. By rebooting and rebalancing the body's metabolism, you can bring your weight into balance and recover vibrant health.

What Exactly Is a Perfect Metabolism?

Let's start with the word **metabolism**. It gets tossed around a lot, but do we really know what it means? What does the metabolism do? Do we have any control over it?

Metabolism is defined as the sum total of all chemical processes that occur in all living organisms to create and sustain life. These chemical reactions control the delivery of material into cells, energy use and production, growth and reproduction, digestion, elimination of waste, and . . . our weight. Our metabolism protects the body from illness and disease as well as playing a role in healing and repair. When all the different processes in the metabolism are working well together, it is called *homeostasis*, which means balance or equilibrium.

Now let's turn to **perfect**. *Perfect* is defined as nothing lacking from the whole, complete.

You might bristle or get defensive at the word *perfect*. Trying to be perfect is an impossible standard, right? We are only human! But that is just one way to look at the word. In this context, *perfect* means whole, complete, holistic. By taking a *holistic* look at the metabolism, we can affect more than just our weight; we address our overall health too.

"The Whole Is Greater than the Sum of Its Parts"

The Gestalt theory of psychology is based on the concept that the human mind as a whole is more complex than just the parts it is composed of. Similarly, our metabolism is based on the interdependence and reliance of different systems—if one is not working right, the whole thing can come crashing down, kind of like dominoes. This concept is sometimes also referred to as *synergy*: one system cannot function optimally without the other.

Western medicine has traditionally been broken into specialties. We see a gastroenterologist for digestive issues, a cardiologist for our heart, and a neurologist for our brain. The upside is that doctors can become experts in their areas. But one downside is that synergies in the body can sometimes be overlooked. Eastern, integrative and functional medicine views the human body as an interconnected whole, with nutrition playing a key role.

The cool thing about taking a nutritional approach to health is that foods are naturally synergistic. Nutrients can magnify the effects of each other, balance each other out, and affect the body holistically. For example, omega-3 fatty acids not only boost our brain function and our mood, but also reduce inflammation and the risk of many diseases. Charlotte Gerson of the famed Gerson Institute put it beautifully:

> *You can't keep one disease and heal two others. When the body heals, it heals everything.*

Weight Is a Symptom

More often than not, when we experience a symptom of some physical imbalance, we go to the doctor or pharmacy to take it away. But our symptoms are clues about what is happening at a deeper level. Our weight is no exception. Being overweight is *just one* of the body's many ways of telling us that our metabolism is off. Other symptoms of an imbalanced metabolism can include elevated triglycerides, cholesterol, and blood sugar levels; fatigue; and cravings/hunger.

When our metabolism is optimized, our weight and many health aspects can come into balance. A healthy metabolism instructs the body to:

- ❦ Properly digest and assimilate nutrients and deliver them to the cells.
- ❦ Effectively eliminate waste materials and toxins and repair damaged cells.
- ❦ Lower elevated blood sugar levels, convert stored fat into fuel, and deliver the energy into the cells.
- ❦ Age gradually and appropriately.
- ❦ Resist and repair viruses and bacteria, and support healing and recovery.
- ❦ Help the body to maintain homeostasis.

Your metabolism could need a reboot if you ever find yourself wondering:

- ❦ Why did everything change when I turned forty? I am eating the same stuff, but I have this *belly*. I just can't seem to button any of my pants anymore!

- Why did it take me two months to lose seven pounds, but only two weeks to gain it all back and then some?

- Why can't I lose any weight around my midsection? I have been working out like a madwoman!

- Why can't I walk up a flight of stairs without getting winded? I just don't seem to have the energy I used to.

- Why do so many foods bother my digestion?

- Do I have arthritis? I'm only thirty-eight, but I have such stiff and achy joints.

- Why does my colleague (who is also fifty years old) look like she is in her early forties, but I look like I am pushing sixty? I don't even recognize myself in the mirror anymore!

- Could I have early dementia? My brain is so foggy, last week I missed two appointments, lost my phone, and forgot to pick up my kids.

- Why can't I seem to make it through the afternoon without a pick-me-up (candy, caffeine, carbs)?

- Why am I so moody and irritable if I don't eat every two hours?

- Why is my blood sugar at 105, when I barely eat any sugary foods? (Anything over ninety puts you in the danger zone, and 100–125 is considered prediabetic.)

- Why am I hungry all the time?

- Why is it so hard to wake up and get out of bed every morning? I need two to three cups of coffee to even function.

- Why can't I fall or stay asleep at night, even when I'm totally exhausted?

- What is causing all my unexplained health issues? In the last five years I have developed fibromyalgia, migraines, arthritis, hypothyroidism, and IBS. I literally feel like I am falling apart!

- Why are my moods so unstable? Could I be depressed?

- Why do I sometimes feel the urge to stop in for a burger, fries, and a shake after a full meal?

All of these questions and other concerns can point to the cascading dominoes of an imbalanced metabolism. The greater the number of symptoms you can relate to, the more out of balance your metabolism could be, and the more dominoes may have fallen.

The bad news is our metabolism tends to slow down as we age due to a number of factors, including nutrition choices, stress, environmental toxins, digestion issues, and undiagnosed food intolerances. But this is also the good news! Many of these factors are in our control, and by changing them with the right information and tools, we can reset our metabolism. The Perfect Metabolism Plan is designed to give you the information and tools you need to make the necessary lifestyle changes and help you to get your metabolism working again.

Three Fundamentals for Change

I hope you are excited to find out how to reboot your metabolism and take back control of your weight and health.

Make no mistake. Change isn't easy. We find comfort in our habits and routines. Many of us have tried to lose weight or change habits and failed on more than one occasion, and we want to avoid feeling that way again. I have found over the years that people don't change without these three fundamentals:

1. You need good information: *The WHAT*.
2. You have to really want it: *The WHY*.
3. You need the tools to make it happen: *The HOW*.

The Perfect Metabolism Plan as outlined in this book delivers them all: Part One is The WHAT: The *Ten Keys* you need to unlock your broken metabolism and break free from calorie-counting and dieting for good! Plus a bonus chapter on timing.

Part Two describes a set of tools to help you to make it happen—The HOW. You will be guided through a gentle, three-phase, foods-based cleanse and elimination diet, designed to help you reboot your metabolism—complete with recipes for highly nourishing and delicious meals. *You can also find more fabulous recipes at www.perfectmetabolism.com.*

The WHY is scattered throughout the entire book to help you identify and connect with your personal motivation.

Please remember that the Perfect Metabolism Plan is not a diet or a get-skinny-quick juice fast. It is about changing your relationship with food to break free from dieting and calorie-counting and find a new way of eating and living that is right for you and your metabolism for the long haul (*no more yo-yo dieting!*).

MINDFUL TIP #1: *LOSE THE GUILT!*

You can't get good results from bad information.

I experienced a lot of guilt as an overweight child. Why couldn't I be a normal size? Why could my siblings eat one piece of grandma's fudge, while I ended up eating eight? I frequently lost control around food and would feel remorseful afterward. I thought I was weak or lazy. Now I know that it was my metabolism. *And yes, even children can suffer from metabolism imbalances and the related diseases. Diseases once called "adult-onset" are affecting increasing numbers of kids today.*

So let's look at the facts so we can move past any guilty feelings you might have saddled yourself with:

- ❧ Much of the nutrition advice you've been given over the years is wrong.

- ❧ That bad information has *crossed your metabolic wires* and messed up your hunger hormones.

You didn't fail . . . your diet failed you!

So how can you stay a healthy weight if your metabolism is not whole? It is next to impossible if you are operating on bad information! So it is time to move past that unearned guilt.

One of the reasons that I am so passionate about sharing the information in this book is because I have struggled with food intolerances, digestive issues, weight imbalances, and more. Let me share my personal health struggles and journey with you.

My Beautiful Health Puzzle—*My Story*

As with many Americans today, my health issues began early. When I was a child, I missed a lot of school because of allergies, recurring ear infections, and digestive trouble. A very picky eater, I started gaining weight in elementary school. By the time I was in sixth grade, I weighed more than I do today. Kids at school picked on me every day for being "chubby." My parents sought out professional help in trying to encourage me to slim down. I can vividly remember making myself a big juicy peanut butter and jelly sandwich before one appointment, kind of like an alcoholic's last drink before heading into rehab! Despite my parents' efforts and continual urging, nothing seemed to work. I just did not want to lose the weight more than I wanted the cookies, ice cream, and PB&Js. The cravings always won.

But then, shortly after I started junior high, things changed. I decided that I didn't want to be called "Chubby Gut" any more. At that moment, my powerful motivation tipped the balance against my cravings. I was able to lose the excess weight, and I went from "Chubby Gut" to "cute" teenager. I think this must have convinced me that being "skinny" was the goal—a mentality that headed me down the wrong path for years. Instead of looking to nurture my body from within, I was focusing on the exterior. I made a lot of mistakes along the way: drinking diet sodas, falling into the low-fat/calorie-cutting trap, trying to go vegetarian (I didn't know what I was doing!), exercising intensely, and still eating lots of sugar.

In my twenties, although I had my weight under control, I was starting to burn out but didn't know it. I was experiencing inflammation, chronic pain, puffiness, frequent sinus infections, foggy thinking, and fatigue. I lost count of the times I was put on antibiotics, and I thought nothing of popping Advil all the time. What I didn't know then was that my symptoms were clues to what was happening deeper within.

I learned that I had Raynaud's disease and a positive ANA (antinuclear antibody)—two indicators of an autoimmune condition (where the body attacks its own cells). Still one symptom shy of a true diagnosis for an autoimmune disorder, I was told it was critical to keep my stress levels down because stress is a "switch" that can turn on disease. I nodded my head vigorously in agreement, yet I had no clue I was even under stress, never mind what I needed to do to control it. I was not aware that my body was under siege from relying on sugar, caffeine, and carbs to keep me going throughout the day. I had no idea that hidden food intolerances and intense cardio workouts were compounding the havoc. My body and adrenals were slowly starting to crash, but I wasn't ready to admit that all the symptoms I was experiencing could be related to diet or lifestyle . . . yet.

By my late thirties, I was still plagued by fatigue, foggy brain, sinus trouble, and chronic aching joints. I was buying Advil in bulk. At one of my many doctor visits, I learned that I had a very low white blood cell count. Looking back at my old records revealed that it had been low for years. My doctor sent me back to the rheumatologist, who ran a battery of tests, and although the ANA marker was still positive, the rest of the tests were negative. I was sent on my way and told again to keep my stress under control. I was relieved to not have lupus but still clueless about why there were so many missing pieces to my health puzzle.

Researching my symptoms, I learned about gluten. Could this be the missing factor? My allergist ran a celiac test. The results were negative, so he told me I could still eat wheat and gluten. (*At the time, virtually no one knew about gluten sensitivity.*) So I did. And I kept popping those Advil.

A turning point came a couple years later when I was introduced to chia seeds. Just adding this one superfood to my daily diet brought big results: soon I had more energy, fewer muscle and joint aches, better digestion, and less of a foggy brain. After more research and despite my negative celiac test, I decided to try going gluten-free. What did I have to lose? It turns out, a lot! I got rid of my puffiness and foggy brain, leveled out my moods, and my chronic aches and pains were fading. Soon I noticed that my seasonal allergies and chronic sinus trouble were not bothering me anymore! Like so many other people, I had assumed that the myriad of symptoms I was experiencing was just "normal" for me and I just had to live with them. I was thrilled to see them gradually disappear. It was then that I knew that I had to learn more about the healing power of foods. I got my nutritionist certification, started up my practice, and soon after created my Perfect Metabolism group program to help others use food to heal too.

This might sound strange, but I am grateful for my health issues. Without them, I would not be where I am today. I am stronger and more whole now because of the path I have been on to heal my own issues. I am more motivated to stay healthy because I know what it feels like to be on the other side.

There is an art form known as *kintsugi,* meaning "golden joinery" through which broken pieces of china are joined together using a golden lacquer. These works are designed not to hide but rather to enhance imperfections. *Kintsugi* thus creates from broken vessels something new and even more beautiful and valuable than the original. It is all about history, transformation, and reinvention. I view my own personal health journey kind of like *kintsugi*—the cracks in my early life have made me perfect in the most imperfect way. It is because of those cracks that I have discovered the golden joinery of fixing our metabolism. I am stronger than ever before and so passionate about spreading the word.

Those cracks happen for everyone—they are simply a part of life. But perhaps the Perfect Metabolism Plan can be the golden glue to help you bring together the pieces and create something new, improved, and transformed.

Your Beautiful Health Puzzle

I encourage you to take a moment and write down your health story. Getting it on paper can help you really connect to your personal motivation for embarking on this change. Maybe along the way, you too will find the missing pieces to your health puzzle that can help you achieve a healthy weight and vibrant health. Looking back at your story at the end of the program can also show you how far you have come and how quickly!

Stop Trying to Lose Weight

This might sound crazy, but I believe that one key to being a healthy weight is to stop focusing on losing weight. As a child, I was told all the time that I had to lose weight. I thought the goal was to be "skinny." For most of my life I had it all wrong. What I finally realized is that our weight and how we look on the outside make up just one indicator of health—and not always a reliable one. In some cases, people who appear "thin" can be as unhealthy as their chubbier counterparts.

I dislike the word *skinny*, and I don't think people should strive to be skinny, nor should we ever refer to people as skinny. But "skinny fat" accurately describes the problem of people who appear to be a healthy weight, but have the same disease markers as their obese counterparts such as high blood pressure, diabetes, etc. According to one 2008 study, one-quarter of all normal weight people fall into this "skinny fat" category. So you see, being a healthy weight does not necessarily mean we are healthy.

If skinny is not the goal, then what is?

Health. It is as simple as that.

Here is the big secret I took almost forty years to figure out: *how our body feels and functions on the inside eventually shows up on the outside.* So if we are eating lots of sugar, drinking too much wine and coffee, skipping meals, and working out to stay thin, those bad habits are going to surface in our health story and in how we feel. If we don't pay for our metabolism imbalances in excess weight, something else will present itself. Often our skin can show the clues of redness, ruddiness, acne, rashes, wrinkles, sagging, puffiness. Or maybe we pay for it with fatigue, joint pain and inflammation, another chronic issue, or worse—it can be allowed to progress to disease.

Assessing Your Progress and Success

I also want you to think about how you want to feel at the end of this. Otherwise how will you know if the Perfect Metabolism Plan worked for you? Ask yourself what you want out of this program:

- ❑ Improved energy or mood?
- ❑ A reduced risk of disease?
- ❑ More energy and less brain fog throughout the day?
- ❑ To get rid of achy joints or digestive issues?
- ❑ To sleep better?
- ❑ To stop cravings?
- ❑ To lose weight?
- ❑ Something else?

If your goal is to reach a healthy weight, one obvious way to assess your success is by weighing and measuring yourself. Readers are encouraged to record their weight and waist measurement at the beginning of the program and again at the end—or weekly if you prefer. I discourage daily weighing because shorter-term fluctuations can be due to changes in water weight and can create an unhealthy focus on the scale. Always remember that weight is just one piece of the health picture. Having some before-and-after blood work done can also allow you to see your markers for disease risk. Visit *www.perfectmetabolism.com* for a list of labs to request from your doctor to identify more quantifiable and measurable results.

Part One

The Ten Keys to Unlocking
Your Perfect Metabolism

Break Up with Sugar
Stop Burning Sugar and Start Burning Fat

Some of the largest companies are now using brain scans to study how we react neurologically to certain foods, especially to sugar. They've discovered that the brain lights up for sugar the same way it does for cocaine.

—MICHAEL MOSS, *Sugar, Salt, Fat: How the Food Giants Hooked Us*

Ahhhh sugar. Sweet, sweet sugar. Sugar tastes good and makes us happy. We reward and comfort ourselves with sweets. Sugar is always there to lift us up when we are down. Sugar shows up for us at every celebration from our first birthday on. So why would I be asking you to give it up? It's no accident that the first Perfect Metabolism Key is *Break Up with Sugar*. It is simply not possible to reach optimal health and metabolism if your blood sugar is not under control.

Sugar gives us a rush of energy, but each rush is followed by a crash. So naturally, we will reach for more sugar to boost our energy and make us "happy" again. I call this cycle the "sugar roller coaster." Being on this ride for too long can wreak havoc on our metabolism and immune system.

Sugar's Dark Side

I always knew sugar wasn't a health food. But I used to think that it was just "empty calories"—not great, but not exactly too bad. Boy was I wrong! The truth is that sugar has a very serious dark side.

As our intake of sugar has steadily increased in the past several decades, so have the rates of obesity and many related diseases. This is not a coincidence! Chronically elevated blood sugar is linked to an increased risk of many—actually *most*—major diseases.

In the short term, diets high in sugar and processed carbohydrates can result in increased hunger/cravings, lowered immunity, mood swings, low energy, acne, and even our looking older. But in the long term, poorly controlled blood sugar is associated with many health issues including an increased risk of heart disease, diabetes, stroke, cancer, liver disease, hormone imbalances, Alzheimer's disease, and more. A study published in *JAMA* in 2014 linked sugar consumption to an increased risk of death, in both normal and overweight individuals. Those whose diet was 25 percent added sugars had more than double the risk of dying from a coronary event. Nope, it's certainly not all sweet when it comes to sugar.

We Need to Get Out of Sugar-Burning Mode

Here's the thing: When we say we want to lose weight, what we really mean is that we want to lose fat. In order to do that, we need to get the body out of *sugar-burning* mode and into *fat-burning* mode. That can only happen if we stop delivering a continual supply of sugar.

Sugar (glucose) supplies immediate energy to our cells. Our metabolism can also convert fat to fuel, but as long as we are supplying it with sugar and simple ("fast") carbs, that will be the primary fuel. When our body is stuck in sugar-burning mode, we are storing more fat than we are burning.

Signs that you could be a "sugar burner":

- Being overweight, especially around the belly/midsection
- A need to eat frequently, or you will suffer from low blood sugar—do you get *hangry* (*angry* when you are *hungry*)?
- Mood swings, anxiety, depression
- Need for caffeine, carbs, and sugar to get you through the day
- Elevated blood glucose or insulin levels, insulin resistance, or diabetes
- Sugar/carb cravings
- Sagging or wrinkled skin—*not aging as gracefully as you'd like*
- Elevated liver enzymes (can be an indicator of fatty liver disease)
- Elevated triglycerides and other heart disease risks

The thing about being in sugar-burning mode is that it turns your metabolism into a stubborn toddler. No matter what (stomp, stomp), it is going to burn sugar! So if there is no sugar available, it might resort to converting protein or breaking down muscle to convert into sugar (*one sign that this might be happening is having thin legs and a big belly*).

In order to get the metabolism working again, we need to retrain the body to use fat as fuel. This means that we need to *significantly* cut back on sugar and simple carbs.

The trouble is most people have no idea that they are getting too much sugar and "fast carbs."

"I Don't Eat Much Sugar"

I hear this all the time. Despite the fact that sugar consumption has sky-rocketed, most people grossly underestimate the amount they consume each day for four main reasons:

1. They are unaware just how much sugar is hidden in the foods they eat and how it all adds up each day.

2. They don't know how much sugar is "too much."

3. They are consuming too many high glycemic foods (many of which can even be low sugar or "healthy" whole grain foods).

4. They are consuming artificial sweeteners, which are as bad as (or worse than) actual sugar for our metabolism.

Let's take a closer look at our sugar sources . . .

1. Hidden Sugars

Because sugar is added to so many foods, we often have no idea how much we are really eating and how quickly it adds up. Food manufacturers are smart; they know people love sugar, so if they want people to buy their product, they just need to make it sweet, right? In fact, the sweeter the food, the better it sells. The more packaged and processed foods you eat, the more added sugar in your diet. According to Dr. Mark Hyman, author of *The Blood Sugar Solution*, "There are 600,000 processed food items in our environment, and 80% of them contain added sugar."

Even people who reach for *seemingly* healthy options are often getting a lot more added sugar than they realize because even foods touted as "healthy" can have loads of sugar.

Some common sources of hidden sugars:

- whole grain cereals and breads
- bars (breakfast, fiber, and protein)
- fruit juices and drinks
- sweetened iced teas and other bottled drinks
- yogurts
- muffins
- coffee drinks (venti mocha latte anyone?)
- condiments
- salad dressings
- marinades
- sauces
- instant oatmeals
- wine, beer, and other alcoholic beverages

It's easy to spot most of the sugar on a food label. If an ingredient ends in -ose (as in sucrose or glucose), it is a form of sugar. But there are other sneaky names that sugar can be hiding behind (some natural and others not so much). Here are some of them: agave, agave nectar, barley malt, beet sugar, brown rice syrup, brown sugar, cane juice, cane juice solids, cane juice crystals, coconut palm sugar, confectioner's sugar, corn sugar, corn syrup, corn syrup solids, caramel, carob syrup, date sugar, dehydrated cane juice, dextrin, dextran, dextrose, diatase, diatastic malt, fructose, fruit juice, fruit juice concentrate, dehydrated fruit juice, fruit juice crystals, glucose, golden syrup, high fructose corn syrup, honey, malt syrup, maltodextrin, maple syrup, palm sugar, palm syrup, powdered sugar, refiner's syrup, sorghum syrup, sucrose, turbinado.

Look for another option if:

- Sugar (in any form) is one of the first two ingredients.

- There are several different types of sugar used (this is often an attempt to disguise sugar).
- High fructose corn syrup is used.

2. Exactly How Much Sugar Is Too Much?

A century ago Americans consumed about forty-five grams of sugar over a five-day period (roughly the amount in one can of soda). Today, we consume about 576 grams of sugar every five days (about equal to seventeen cans of soda)! That adds up to over 130 pounds of sugar a year! Teenage boys are getting the most—*over 500 calories of sugar a day.*

Even if we track how much sugar we are really eating every day, we still might not know how much is too much. Recommended guidelines do exist, but they are not widely disseminated. Because of the powerful link between sugar and heart disease, not surprisingly, the American Heart Association (AHA) recommends limiting *added sugars* to no more than about 6–7 percent of total calories each day. (Added sugars are those put in during processing of foods, such as sugar-sweetened cereals, or supplements we make at serving, such as the sugar you stir into a cup of tea.) This means that on average, women should have no more than six teaspoons (twenty-four grams) of added sugars a day. Men should get no more than nine teaspoons (thirty-six grams) on average daily. Given that one twelve-ounce soda or bottled coffee drink generally has about ten teaspoons, holding this line may not be so easy.

Figure out how much sugar you are getting each day. Do the math to determine the sugar content of foods: 4 grams of sugar = 1 teaspoon of sugar. Just divide the grams by four to get the number of teaspoons per serving. A product that has twelve grams of sugar per serving, will have three teaspoons of sugar per serving.

As we know, sugar is lurking in so many foods, even "healthy" options.

- one fruit-on-the-bottom yogurt: 26 grams (6 tsp)—*some of which are naturally occurring*
- instant apple cinnamon oatmeal cup: 20 grams (5 tsp)

See how easy it is to shatter the recommended limits for sugar before the clock strikes noon—even when we are making "healthy choices"? Grab a bottled iced coffee and you surpass another day's limit: 46 grams (11 tsp)!

It can be eye-opening to add up all the added sugar you get in a day's time—make sure to count everything—candies, dressings, sauces, and more.

3. High Glycemic Foods—Are Pretzels Worse Than a Candy Bar?

Here is the kicker: sugar isn't the whole story. Foods don't need to be sweet to spike our blood sugar. In fact, many of the foods that send our blood sugar soaring the highest are actually low-sugar foods. You might be thinking, "Wait, how could a low-sugar food affect my blood sugar?" To understand that, let's take a look at the glycemic index.

The Glycemic Index—What Is It?

Our bodies convert the foods that we eat into usable energy for our cells. All carbohydrates (whether in the form of a candy bar, a piece of toast, a handful of pretzels, or one of those 100-calorie snack packs) get converted to sugar, a usable energy form for the body.

The "glycemic index" is the measure for how fast and how much a carbohydrate gets converted to sugar. Foods are given a number between 1 and 100 (or higher in some cases). The lower a food is on the glycemic index, the more gradually it increases blood sugar and/or to a lower level. The higher the glycemic number, the faster and/or higher that food will spike the blood sugar:

- High glycemic: 70 and above
- Medium glycemic: 56–69
- Low glycemic: Under 55

When we eat a lot of high glycemic foods, our blood sugar spikes higher and faster. Doing this all day long is a recipe for a metabolism meltdown, which raises our risk for many diseases. Research out of Harvard has demonstrated that eating more low glycemic foods can lower the risks for obesity and related conditions like coronary heart disease and diabetes.

A sampling of foods and their glycemic indexes, according to Harvard Health Publications

- Gatorade 78
- Colas 63

- Milk 32
- Ice cream 57
- Yogurt, fruit 36
- Corn flakes 93
- Frosted Flakes 55
- Oatmeal 55
- Instant oatmeal 83
- Baked russet potato 111
- Doughnut 76
- Pretzels 83
- Snickers candy bar 51
- Table sugar 64
- Maltose 105
- Honey 62
- Fructose 22
- Apple 39
- Grapes 46
- Raisins 64
- Watermelon 72
- French bread, baguette 95
- White bagel 72
- Whole wheat bread 71 (average)

Not All Sugars Are Processed the Same

One of the reasons that colas are below 70 on the glycemic index has to do with the fact that most sodas contain high fructose corn syrup—which is made up of both fructose and glucose. Fructose is processed differently than glucose and most other sugars. Because fructose does not require insulin to get into the cells, it is lower on the glycemic index and was originally thought to be a healthier option. But it is primarily processed in the liver, and research is linking *excess* fructose consumption to elevated triglycerides and even nonalcoholic fatty liver disease. The majority of excess fructose consumed generally comes from drinking sodas sweetened with high fructose corn syrup.

Are Pretzels Worse than a Candy Bar?

You might have noticed that pretzels (as well as baked potatoes, wheat bread, and corn flakes) are quite high on the glycemic index, despite being low-sugar foods. How could a low-sugar food like pretzels spike our blood sugar higher than a doughnut or a cola? White potatoes and foods made from flours and enriched processed grains—like crackers, breads, and pretzels—are converted very quickly into sugar when they enter our bloodstream. That is how they spike our blood sugar levels, cause insulin to be released, and as a result, make our appetite increase. Let's take a closer look.

Ahhhh pretzels. I used to think pretzels were the perfect snack: they only had one gram of sugar, so that meant they are healthy, right? I munched on them every afternoon. I needed them; rather, I was addicted to them. I can even remember stopping to buy them when I traveled out of town. But now I know pretzels were one of "*my sugars*," because they were spiking my blood sugar to eighty-three every time I ate them. I call simple carbs like pretzels "appetite stimulants" because they don't satisfy. They make you hungrier and cause you to crave more sugar and carbs. It's no wonder I used to go through several bags of them every week.

In order to get your blood sugar under control, you should be conscious of the glycemic index of foods. Foods with a higher glycemic index are sometimes referred to as "fast carbs," because they spike your blood sugar faster and higher. Focusing on "slow" or low glycemic carbs is critical to keeping blood sugar on an even keel. Refer to the above list, and find more details at *www.perfectmetabolism.com*.

But What about "Healthy Whole Wheat?"

In stores and restaurants these days, we are seeing "*healthier*" whole wheat versions of so many things—breads, cookies, pastas, pizza crusts, rolls, cereals, etc. We may not like the taste and texture as much, but we choose these options because we are trying to be healthier! And the whole wheat version has fiber and whole grains, so it is better for us, right? Well, fiber generally does keep our blood sugar lower. *That is one reason why eating a whole apple is better for us than drinking apple juice.* But there are several reasons why whole wheat may not be as healthy as we thought. One reason is that even whole wheat bread is a *high glycemic* food. In fact, wheat bread spikes our blood sugar higher than some candy bars.

Many breads labeled "whole wheat" are really made with highly processed *enriched* wheat flour, which doesn't exactly resemble a whole grain anymore. They often contain high fructose corn syrup or multiple types of sugar. Many contain a significant amount of added gluten and even chemical-based dough "conditioners." Here is the ingredient list for a popular brand of hamburger buns labeled "whole wheat" and "heart healthy" on the front:

> *whole wheat flour, water, wheat gluten, high fructose corn syrup, yeast. Contains 2% or less of each of the following: soybean oil, salt, brown sugar, distilled vinegar, calcium sulfate, dough conditioners (may contain one or more of the following: mono- and diglycerides, ethoxylated mono- and diglycerides, sodium stearoyl lactylate, calcium peroxide, datem, ascorbic acid, azodicarbonamide, enzymes), calcium propionate (preservative), yeast nutrients (monocalcium phosphate, calcium sulfate, ammonium sulfate), corn starch, guar gum, natural flavors, vitamin D3, soy lecithin, milk, soy flour, sesame seeds.*

The main ingredient in this bun is flour, not whole grains. The third ingredient is gluten. The fourth ingredient is high fructose corn syrup. It also contains brown sugar. Many commercial breads like this one contain a chemical called azodicarbonamide. This whole wheat bun is hardly a health food; in fact, it is hardly food at all in my opinion! Many of the above ingredients look more like a science experiment than a food!

It is not just the processed whole wheat breads that are causing us trouble. There are several other things about whole wheat that are messing with our metabolism. In the chapter about food intolerances, we will take a closer look at how whole wheat could be wreaking some serious havoc on your metabolism and weight. For now, let's move on to the fourth reason we are getting too much sugar . . .

4. Artificial Sweeteners

They seem like the perfect solution, right? You get to keep the sweetness without the calories. Unfortunately, artificial sweeteners are not that innocent, nor are they good for our waistline. Approximately 200 times sweeter than sugar, chemical sweeteners like aspartame and sucralose can confuse our hunger hormones and stimulate our appetite. Several studies on both rats and humans found that those who consumed artificial sweeteners weighed more than those who did not. Artificial sweeteners may also increase the risk of developing diabetes and metabolic syndrome (a group of risk factors associated with heart disease). Drinking diet sodas was found to be associated with a 44 percent increased risk of heart disease. So in order to boost our metabolism and break free from sugar, we also need to avoid foods and drinks that contain artificial sweeteners.

But that may be easier said than done, right? A lot of Americans are hooked on diet sodas. There was a time when I didn't think a day could go by without my diet sodas. But it is possible to give them up, I promise. And since I dropped them, I have realized they were giving me a wide range of other negative symptoms ranging from headaches to dizziness. Artificial sweeteners are considered "excitotoxic," which means they can overstimulate and damage nerve cells, leading to a negative impact on the brain, nervous system, and other organs. Read the books *Sweet Deception, Sweet Poison* or *Excitotoxins: The Taste that Kills* if you want to learn more about the damaging effects of excitoxins (like aspartame and MSG) on the brain and nervous system.

Here are some nice alternatives to diet drinks:

- Sparkling water with a squeeze of lime or lemon
- "Fancy water"—adding slices of cucumber, lemon, lime, ginger, mint leaves, or apple slices with a cinnamon stick to your fresh filtered water
- Unsweetened iced tea with lemon
- Kombucha tea (a fizzy fermented tea with natural probiotics and B vitamins)—one of my personal favorites!
- Herbal tea with a teaspoon of coconut oil (nips sugar cravings in the bud)
- Bragg Lemonade (see recipes)

The Role of Hormones in Metabolism

When our hormones are not working well, neither is our metabolism. It's kind of like the game *Telephone* we played in elementary school. Everyone sits in a circle, and the first person whispers something to the next person, that person does the same, and so on, until the message gets back to the one who first said it. Along the way, the message often gets mixed up. The original statement might have been "I want peas, meat, and potatoes." But by the end it could be "I want to please meet in the toes." It might sound vaguely similar to the original message, yet the real meaning is totally lost! This is what can happen with our hormones: the messages get sent out, but they are not delivered or received correctly.

Throughout this book, I will be highlighting some of the major hormones that affect our appetite, blood sugar management, blood pressure, and more. Let's take a closer look at the primary hormone that regulates our blood sugar in our first *hormone highlight*.

HORMONE HIGHLIGHT: INSULIN

- **Insulin:** A hormone produced by the pancreas in response to elevated blood sugar. Insulin's job is to get the sugar out of the blood and deliver it to cells to be used for energy. Insulin has another important job—to instruct the body to store excess sugars. Some can be stored in the liver as glycogen, but the vast majority gets stored as adipose tissue or fat.

- **Insulin resistance:** When blood sugar is repeatedly spiked, after a while our body can become resistant to insulin. One analogy would be this situation: Let's say there are 150 people (sugar) in a movie theater with five exits (insulin receptors). The fire alarm goes off. If everything is working well, the moviegoers have five exits to use to move to safety, and the building can be evacuated in a timely manner (*glucose is delivered efficiently to insulin receptors/cells*). But what if three of the exits were stuck shut? Some people would be running around testing doors to find one that works, others would be lined up at the two working doors waiting to leave (*glucose* *is hanging around looking for a receptor because some of the insulin receptors are no longer responding; blood sugar stays elevated longer).* When more moviegoers are stuck inside, more firefighters are sent in to try to get people out of the movie theater (*the pancreas keeps releasing more insulin to try to lower the glucose levels).* Because the exits don't work, the firefighters find a place to put folks where they can be kept safe (*similar to how the body stores the glucose in the fat cells).* The favorite places to store fat are in the midsection and around the organs—which is the most dangerous place for it to be.

How do you know if you have insulin resistance? There are often no obvious symptoms, but these can be a clue:

- Weight gain around the midsection
- Low energy
- Difficulty losing weight
- Dark patches on neck, armpits, and other areas (acanthosis nigricans) *in advanced cases*
- Chronically elevated blood sugar

Two tests that can help identify insulin problems are the A1C and a fasting glucose test. Fasting blood glucose numbers consistently near 100 are troubling and could mean insulin resistance. Between 100 and 125 is classified as prediabetes; over 125 is diabetes. But even "safe" levels of blood sugar (85 mg/dl) are associated with chronic inflammation, insulin resistance, and an increased risk of disease. Ideal fasting glucose levels are between 70 and 85 mg/dl. The A1C measures glycation, which shows the average blood sugar over a longer period, and should ideally be under 5.5. An A1C of 5.7 to 6.4 indicates prediabetes, and results above 6.5 are indicative of diabetes according to the National Diabetes Information Clearinghouse (NDIC). Studies published in the *British Journal of Cancer* have also linked elevated A1C results to increased risk for cancer and dementia. Your doctor might also want to order a glucose tolerance test.

What Is *Your* Sugar?

Sugar is not just the white stuff. It's the wine in the evening, sweets after dinner, pretzels in the afternoon, diet sodas, candies, cereal bars, sweet dressings on your salad, crackers. I'm sure you know which ones are yours.

Like many people, my love affair with sugar began early. Throughout my life, my "sugar" has shifted with my activities. Some of my fondest childhood memories were about sweets—grandma's fudge at Christmas, baking cookies with my sister, trips to the ice cream parlor in the summer, candy and soda at the movies. Later, my sugar was diet sodas, pretzels, a couple of glasses of wine at night, after-dinner sweets, and more. Even though "my sugar" changed as I got older, the addiction carried over.

I cannot overemphasize this: if you want to heal your metabolism, breaking up with sugar is critical. Most people with chronically elevated blood sugar have no idea that they have it. Unless your blood sugar is frequently above 100 mg/dl, your doctor probably won't even mention it. According to the Center for Disease Control, one-third of the population is prediabetic, but those numbers are likely underestimated.

So now is the time to get real with yourself about which sugars you go to and wean yourself off them. One way to do this is to follow the Perfect Metabolism *Rule of Three*.

The Perfect Metabolism Rule of Three

Stabilizing the blood sugar is critical for a healthy metabolism, and for disease prevention. To get out of the sugar-burning mode and into fat-burning mode, I recommend following a Rule of Three for choosing what to eat: include at least one or more of the following three things *each time you eat* to keep your blood sugar stable, hunger hormones in balance, and energy higher. Get more than one of the following, and you will stay satisfied longer and keep your blood sugar more stable:

1. **Protein.** Choose high-quality organic, free-range animal as well as plant-based proteins (nuts, seeds, hemp, chia, quinoa).

2. **Fiber.** Primarily reach for those found in vegetables, seeds, low-sugar whole fruits, nongluten whole grains, etc. Fiber helps to

lower the glycemic response, especially soluble fiber such as that found in chia seeds.

3. **Fat.** Pick healthy fat sources like avocados, coconut, and butter processed from cows that graze on grass. This is becoming easier to find as more consumers are demanding it and as more growers are raising their cattle strictly on the food they were meant to eat). This one is really critical. I can almost guarantee that if you have issues with blood sugar, you are not getting enough of the right fats. Stay tuned, chapter two is dedicated to fats.

Reset Your Sweet Tooth

Eating a lot of super sweet foods over time makes our taste buds less sensitive to sweets. So we need more and more to satisfy our sweet "tooth." This is why taking a vacation from foods that have a lot of added sugars is a good way to reset our sweet tooth and insulin sensitivity. The longer you go without sweets, the less you will crave super sweet foods, and the better your body will get at dealing with them. You might even begin to find some really sweet foods almost repulsive! I used to love a good caramel sundae; now the idea of eating ice cream drenched in sauce is not appealing to me in the least!

Any Good Alternatives?

You will notice that some of the recipes in the Perfect Metabolism Plan include *small amounts* of natural sweeteners like *stevia, raw honey,* or *coconut palm sugar/nectar.* That is because I am a realist and a foodie. I want food to taste good, and I also want you to stick with this and enjoy it. I have found that some recipes and foods need just a hint of sweetness to make them more palatable and enjoyable. But it is important to resist the urge to sweeten foods to what your taste buds are used to; otherwise, you will not *reset your sweet tooth.*

Note: not everyone loves stevia, because it has a slightly bitter aftertaste. One thing that I do is combine a little bit of stevia with another caloric sweetener like coconut palm nectar or raw honey in a recipe. I find that they can balance each other out: stevia reduces the caloric impact, and the natural sweetener reduces the bitterness. Some people also believe that stevia can have an effect similar to artificial sweeteners, confusing the hunger regulatory systems. So using a blend of sweeteners can avoid that issue as well.

What about Fruits?

Sugar occurs naturally in some foods (such as fruit, milk). Because whole fruits also contain fiber, vitamins, minerals, and antioxidants along with the naturally occurring sugars, eating whole, fresh fruit is certainly different from eating candy. In healthy, active individuals, the sugars in whole fruit are generally not concerning. But for those with insulin resistance, high triglycerides, fatty liver, high uric acid levels, or diabetes, eating a lot of higher glycemic fruits can cause blood sugar issues too. So if you want to lose weight on this program, plan to temporarily limit your fruit consumption to no more than one to two small servings (¼–½ cup) of lower-sugar fruits such as berries per day. But if it comes down to choosing between a piece of whole fruit or candy, always go with the whole fresh fruit because it comes paired with fiber, vitamins, and minerals!

Fruit juice, on the other hand, lacks the fiber, and so it will spike the blood sugar higher and faster. Also most prepared juice is pasteurized, which destroys many of the nutrients anyway. So skip the fruit juice. If you do choose a fresh-pressed juice, make sure it is primarily vegetable juice and have it with some chia seeds or a handful of nuts, which will level out the blood sugar and help with the absorption of fat-soluble vitamins. Dried fruit is also something to be cautious about. A concentrated source of natural sugars, dried fruits can create blood sugar surges and stimulate cravings, and many also contain sulfites.

SUGAR AND YEAST OVERGROWTH

People who have very powerful cravings for sugar, carbs, and alcohol or who feel sick when they try to give them up might have something called candida yeast overgrowth. Everyone has some candida yeast in their digestive tract, and as long as there is a healthy balance of good bacteria, the candida yeast should not give us health problems. But if the yeasts are allowed to grow out of control, that is when the candida can wreak havoc on our health. Often a course of antibiotics can be the start of the problem. Antibiotics kill bacteria—the good along with the bad. If we wipe out all the bacteria, that can set the stage for the yeast to take over. Yeasts love sugar. So a diet high in sugars essentially feeds the yeast. A course or two of antibiotics and a diet high in sugar can lead to yeast overgrowth. Symptoms include headaches (mild to mind-blowing), constipation, food intolerances, bladder or vaginal infections, muscle and joint aches, toenail fungus, sinus pain and stuffiness, fatigue, foggy brain—just to name a few.

Those suspecting candida need to be *very strict* about removing all sugars and simple carbs, alcohol, vinegar, corn, and fruit from their diet and will want to make sure to take a high-quality probiotic designed to repopulate the gut with healthy bacteria. *Note:* If initially you feel worse taking a probiotic, it could be some die-off of the yeasts. If you suspect that you have candida, consider finding a qualified health practitioner to diagnose this and any other issues (such as parasites, or a buildup of heavy metals) and support you to recover.

MINDFUL TIP #2:
MOVE BEYOND INSTANT GRATIFICATION TO MINDFUL EATING

I am not going to lie to you—trying to give up sugar can be really difficult. Sugar is addictive. You might need to hit the mental *override button* to get through the first few days.

Do you find that if you sit down in front of a plate of cookies, all of a sudden you have eaten half of them? Maybe it is the chips and dip or the ice cream. Or maybe you go for pretzels and diet sodas like I did. We start with a bite, but we keep going back for more and have soon polished off a pint or a dozen. It is easy to do, because these foods don't satisfy, rather they stimulate our appetite.

When we eat mindlessly, we find ourselves out of control around foods, and then we are left to deal with feelings of guilt.

So instead it is time to . . .

FLIP IT!

Instead of eating mindlessly and then ruminating about it for hours afterward . . .

Think first, then eat.

Before you get something to eat, *pause* and ask yourself:

1. First and foremost, am I really hungry? Or am I:

   ◆ bored?

   ◆ sad?

   ◆ tired?

   ◆ angry?

   ◆ thirsty?

2. If you *are* really hungry, look at what is in front of you and consider this:

   ◆ Will this help to create my Perfect Metabolism or take away from it?

   ◆ Is this something that will make my body and mind feel and function at its best ten minutes, thirty minutes, two hours after I eat it?

   ◆ Is this something that I really want?

This is called "mindful eating." Think beyond the *instant gratification* of how that food *tastes*, and be conscious about how that food will make you *feel*. If you do end up snacking on something that is not ideal—connect back in. How did this make me feel and function? That can help you to be more mindful next time.

A Little Added Support

As you begin to incorporate more fiber, protein, and healthy fats (especially chia seeds and coconut oil) into your diet (see chapter two), you should naturally start to see your cravings diminish. But some people find that they need a little bit of extra support initially. Below are some key foods, herbs, and supplements you might find helpful (always check with your doctor first if you are taking medication or have an existing condition):

1. **Coconut oil.** Known to help in controlling blood sugar and improving the secretion of insulin, coconut oil also aids effective utilization of blood glucose. See chapter two for more about how to use coconut oil to support a healthy metabolism.

2. **Chia seeds.** When properly hydrated, chia seeds fill us up, slow the absorption of sugar into the bloodstream, and help to keep blood sugar level. Read more about this amazing super seed in chapter two.

3. **Probiotics.** Eating a lot of sugar is like sending out an invitation to yeasts and bacteria (the "bad guys") to come to a party in our gut. An overabundance of yeasts can cause sugar cravings and affect our digestion, our weight, our immune system, and so much more. We need to boost the "good guys" to level the playing field. Adding a prebiotic fiber can also help to get the probiotics to colonize the gut. Learn more about probiotics in chapter three. Take a high-quality probiotic each evening before bedtime, *ideally with at least 20 billion live active cultures. See the sidebar about yeast overgrowth, and read more in chapter three.*

4. **Omega-3 fish oils.** Shown to lower inflammation, turn on fat-burning hormones, improve insulin sensitivity, and support mood, a daily high-quality purified fish oil with approximately 500 mg of DHA and 500 mg of EPA is beneficial.

5. **L-glutamine.** Those with powerful sugar and alcohol cravings might benefit from taking the amino acid L-glutamine. According to Julia Ross in *The Diet Cure*, the recommended dose for sugar cravings is generally 500 milligrams (mg) three to four times daily between meals. For really strong cravings, she says you can open a capsule directly onto the tongue. It also supports repair of the gut wall lining, boosts the immune system, and more. L-glutamine can be constipating in some—stop taking it if you have this reaction.

6. **Cinnamon.** Studies show that half a teaspoon of cinnamon can improve insulin sensitivity, help regulate blood sugar levels, and reduce cravings. It also has been shown to improve triglycerides and cholesterol levels. I like to add some to my morning smoothies, chia pudding, etc. *Note:* I recommend getting the Ceylon type, or "true cinnamon." Cassia, the more common kind of cinnamon, contains higher levels of coumarin, which could be toxic to the liver in high amounts. Ceylon cinnamon is a little harder to find, but it is worth it.

7. **Magnesium.** Important for activating the fat-burning hormone adiponectin, magnesium is also known to support healthy blood sugar regulation. Raw cacao, leafy greens, nuts, and seeds are all good food sources. Magnesium needs can vary depending on individual activity levels, stress levels, and alcohol consumption. The RDA is 300–420 mg daily, but many will benefit from higher levels. The best forms are citrate, malate, glycinate, or orotate (not oxide, which is poorly absorbed). Cut back if you get loose stools.

8. **Chromium picolinate.** The human body only needs a small amount of chromium, which is why it is measured in micrograms, not milligrams. Studies show that chromium might be useful for supporting a healthy insulin response and carbohydrate metabolism. A therapeutic dose is generally between 250 and 500 micrograms (mcg), taken once or twice a day. But even doses of 150–250 mcg total per day have been shown to have favorable effects on blood sugar regulation.

9. **B complex vitamins.** Very important for detoxification, cellular energy, sleep, neurotransmitters, the metabolism of sugars, and the production of hormones, B vitamins are depleted under stress and high sugar consumption. In addition to getting quality animal proteins, you might want to take a high quality B complex to keep energy levels up, support detox pathways and the sleep cycle, and boost the metabolism. Some people might benefit from getting a B complex shot; most integrative doctors offer this service *(make sure they use the active methyl form of B12).*

The Bottom Line

It is not easy to give up something as addictive and pervasive as sugar. But I promise you it is possible with the right tools and information, even if you have tried and failed in the past. Making this change will not only boost your metabolism and improve your energy, mood, immunity, overall health; it will also reduce your risk of most major diseases. Keeping blood sugar level is critical to maintaining a healthy weight and metabolism.

Remember the Rule of Three when choosing what foods to eat. Get some fat (healthy kind), fiber, and/or protein (high quality) at each meal or snack.

This book shares several tips and tricks along the way to help you. In chapter two, you will learn all about helpful healthy fats, critical to getting rid of sugar. In part two, you will be led through a gentle food elimination diet and cleanse, supported by recipes for successfully removing sugar from your life . . . for good! I will also share my personal sugar roller-coaster past and guide you to write your *Sugar Breakup Letter*. Stay tuned . . .

✌ 2 ✍

Fix Your Fats!
Healthy Fats Are Critical to a Perfect Metabolism

I had found in my clinical practice that the more good fats people eat, the healthier they become.

—DR. DIANA SCHWARZBEIN, *The Schwarzbein Principle*

Fat Is Not a Four-Letter Word.

For the past few decades, fats have been demonized. Many of us have had the erroneous messages pounded into our heads: "Fat makes us fat." "Fats promote heart disease." "Low-fat is healthy." "Saturated fats and cholesterol clog up arteries." We all dutifully ran out to buy low- and no-fat foods, gobbling them up with relish—because, "They have no fat, so they won't make me fat, right?" I bought it hook, line, and sinker too. I remember eating reduced-fat cookies, fat-free yogurts, and skim milk with everyone else!

But it turns out that fat is not the enemy. In fact, fat is our friend. Fat is critical for a healthy metabolism because it stabilizes our blood sugar, nourishes cell membranes, boosts satiety, improves nutrient absorption, and so much more. Fat-free foods are by definition processed, and often when the fat is removed, it is replaced with sugar, corn syrup solids, and other ingredients that are terrible for us. Even when fat is removed from foods without sugars being added back (such as with skim milk), the *percentage* of sugar and our glycemic response goes up, which means that reduced- and non-fat foods impact our blood sugar more than full-fat foods like whole milk. Research is confirming that reduced-fat foods are not better for us.

Without sufficient healthy fats, our hunger hormones can go haywire. Let's take a quick look back at how this low- and no-fat dogma came about.

The History Behind the Low-Fat Craze

In the early 1900s heart disease was virtually unheard of, occurring in only about 1 percent of the population. But by 1921, it had become the leading cause of death in the United States! How could this possibly happen? A researcher named Dr. Ancel Keys believed that cholesterol and saturated fat intake were to blame for the heart disease epidemic, so he set out to prove his theory. After presenting his initial study and hypothesis at a World Health Organization meeting, he was ridiculed. So he went back to the drawing board and looked at data from around the world to identify a link between fat intake and heart disease. He then released his Seven Countries Study, which reported that a high intake of saturated fat and cholesterol indeed correlated with a higher risk of heart disease.

But there were two very serious flaws with the Seven Countries Study. The first was that it was based on *correlation*, not *causation*. Without identifying causation, we can't be sure that another factor wasn't the *real* cause of the heart disease epidemic. Perhaps, say, sugar or starch intake? In fact, some of Keys's critics believed that sugar was one of the main reasons for the heart disease epidemic. The second serious flaw is where the story starts to get interesting. Despite being named the *Seven* Countries Study, Keys had examined data from twenty-two countries. So why did he only report data from seven? Some of the other countries disproved his theory because they showed an inverse relationship between cholesterol, saturated fat, and heart disease! Despite these flaws, the American Heart Association took notice of Keys's research and informed the public in 1956 that consuming saturated fats and cholesterol was associated with a higher risk of heart disease. Keys even graced the cover of *Time* magazine in 1961. Later, largely based on Keys's work, the USDA published nutrition recommendations urging Americans to reduce their intake of fat and cholesterol and eat more grains and carbs.

The history continues. Another famous study started in 1948, the Framingham Heart Study, was designed to identify factors contributing to cardiovascular disease. This ongoing study found no correlation between cholesterol intake and heart disease. The researchers were so puzzled with the findings that the results were unfortunately not published. Meanwhile, for more than a half a century, Americans have been dutifully following the recommendations to eat a "heart-healthy" low-fat diet!

Since the 1980s the incidence of diabetes has tripled from 5.6 million to over 20 million (CDC). It is predicted that one in three people will have diabetes by the year 2050 if something does not stop this trajectory. One out of every 4 deaths is now due to heart disease. Between the years 1960 and 1995, the consumption of dietary fats dropped from 40 percent of the diet to 33 percent, while consumption of carbs went from 45 percent to 52 percent. In the early 1900s, sugar consumption was about two teaspoons a day; now it has skyrocketed to over twenty-five—which adds up to about 150 pounds annually! Just in the last thirty years sugar consumption has increased by about thirty pounds annually.

The French Paradox

Meanwhile over in France, they have enjoyed pâté, quiche, and liberally used butter and crème fraiche. The French in general are a healthy weight. This has been commonly referred to as "the French Paradox," because based on our knowledge at the time, a low-fat diet was supposedly better for our weight and health. It turns out that it really isn't a paradox at all: the French had it right all along. Eating a high-quality diet with healthy fats is probably one of the key reasons that the French *don't* tend to struggle with weight gain.

The real truth is that *healthy fats do not make you fat.* In fact, it is almost impossible to be a healthy weight unless you get enough healthy fat in your daily diet.

Fats Are Essential for Life!

If you are trying to avoid fats, it is not surprising that you might be craving them. Fats are essential for life! Critical for healthy hormones, fats (lipids) help us to feel satiated and keep our moods and blood sugar stable. Fats and cholesterol make up about 60 percent of the structure of our brains and are also found in our skin, hair, cells, and blood. They play an important role in our cellular structure and functioning, as well as regulation of our hormones and metabolism, brain function, nutrient absorption, reproductive health, vision/eye health, skin, heart health, and more.

But wait: before you run to the store and buy up a bunch of ice cream, cakes, and pies with abandon, realize that not all fats are the same.

Not All Fats Are Created Equal

Saturated fats and cholesterol have been given a bad rap as the "fall guys" in the heart disease epidemic over the past couple decades. But to say that all saturated fats and cholesterol are bad is very misguided. A meta-analysis of studies published in the *American Journal of Clinical Nutrition* looked at almost 350,000 cases and found that there was "no significant evidence that dietary saturated fat is associated with an increased risk of coronary heart disease." Saturated fats are not bad for us; in fact our cells need a balance of both unsaturated and saturated fatty acids—and yes even cholesterol—in order to function optimally.

However, there is one common denominator that determines if a fat is bad for us, and that is if it is damaged or oxidized. These fats lead to metabolism problems and disease. How do fats become damaged? By being exposed to high heat, as in processing and frying, as well as by altering the fats, as in trans fats.

Let's look at a breakdown of the types of fat:

- **Saturated fats** are highly stable, which means they are less likely to get damaged, oxidized, or go rancid. Even when cooked at medium to high heats, most saturated fats tend to remain stable. This is an important advantage, as consuming damaged and rancid fats can be very harmful to our health. Saturated fats also provide needed stability to our cells. Animal fats such as butter and lard contain between 40 and 60 percent saturation, which interestingly enough very closely matches the profile of human cells, which are about 50 percent saturated too. Ghee (clarified butter) is one of the best cooking oils, because it is stable up to 485 degrees and very healing to the digestion. Look for grass-fed or pasture-raised butter, because it contains conjugated linoleic acid (CLA), linked to a reduction in body fat accumulation. Up to 90 percent saturated, coconut oil is a very unique fat with amazing properties for our metabolism and overall health. *See more about the benefits of coconut oil later under My Favorite Fats.*

- **Unsaturated fats** provide flexibility to our cellular structure. There are two types of unsaturated fats:

    - **Monounsaturated fats** are liquid at room temperature and also fairly stable, which means that, like saturated fats, they are less likely to become damaged. Olives and avocados contain a high amount of monounsaturated fatty acids. Extra virgin olive oil is stable at low to medium temperatures, so it is best used on raw foods or at low to medium heats. Virgin olive oil is stable under 420 degrees. Avocado oil has one of the highest smoking points of all fats, so it can be used for high-heat cooking (up to 500 degrees), but it also is a wonderfully versatile oil to be used raw, such as in dressings and pestos.

◆ **Polyunsaturated fats** are also liquid at room temperature even when refrigerated, which is one reason they are often used in salad dressings. Because polyunsaturated fats are unstable, just the processing and bottling of polyunsaturated fats can cause them to become damaged or rancid because of the high heats involved. Another way they can become damaged is during cooking, especially at high heats. So if you do choose to use occasionally a polyunsaturated oil, make sure to select the cold-pressed variety, which means neither heat nor chemicals were used to extract the oil.

One group of polyunsaturated fats—the omegas—are considered "essential fatty acids" because they must be obtained from the diet:

❋ Omega-3 fats are found in fatty fish, some nuts, seeds, algae, grass-fed meats, and pastured chicken eggs. *Omega-3s reduce inflammation in the body.*

❋ Omega-6 fats are abundant in the American diet because they are found in polyunsaturated vegetable oils and products made with them. Conventionally raised animal proteins ("feedlot farmed") also have higher concentrations of omega-6s than omega-3s, which makes them more inflammatory. *Omega-6s increase inflammation.*

❋ Having the right balance of omega fatty acids is important for preventing inflammation: we should be getting a 1:3 ratio of omega-3s to omega-6s in our diets. But because most processed foods are made with oils that are high in omega-6s (i.e., cheap soy, cottonseed, or vegetable oils), we are often taking in closer to a 1:20 ratio. This sets us up for chronic inflammation (read more about the omegas and inflammation in chapter six).

Avoid This Fat Like the Plague

There is one type of fat that should be shunned at all costs: trans fat. Trans fats occur naturally in small amounts in some animal products, which is not concerning. The majority of trans fats in our diets are manufactured fats, which are highly damaged fats. Linked to many health problems, trans fats raise triglycerides, inflammation, and LP(a) (the dense and more damaging kind of LDL cholesterol) and also may make blood platelets stickier. Trans fats are produced by partially hydrogenating a fat, which changes it from a liquid to a solid at room temperature. Trans fats extend the shelf life of a product cheaply, so it is no surprise that food manufacturers might want to use them. But the FDA recently moved to ban them and has now required that labels list them. Be sure to read labels carefully because as long as a product has less than 0.5 grams of trans fats, the label can say "zero trans fats." However, we often eat more than one serving of these foods, so they can quickly add up. And no amount of trans fats is safe. Look for *partially hydrogenated oils* among the ingredients. If these words appear, the food contains trans fats. Even *fully hydrogenated* can mean there are trans fats. It is ironic that margarine used to be recommended as a healthier option to butter because stick margarines have plentiful trans fatty acids. Trans fats also hide in a long list of "convenience foods": coffee creamers, fried foods, frozen dinners, microwave popcorn, commercial baked goods, canned frosting, frozen soft serve treats, and refrigerated dough for cookies, piecrusts, and biscuits.

Fats + Carbs = Good or Bad?

Because fats help to keep the blood sugar level and create a feeling of longer-lasting satiety, it would make sense that eating some fat with carbohydrates is useful in keeping the blood sugar levels more stable, right?

Let's look at some facts:

1. Eating sugar and carbs causes blood sugar to spike, so the pancreas releases insulin to pull the glucose from the blood and deliver it as energy to the cells.

2. The presence of insulin is a signal to the body to store fat, especially in the midsection.

3. Eating fats does not stimulate the release of insulin, so healthy fats are less likely to lead to fat storage when eaten on their own.

4. If we eat fat *along with* the sugar or high glycemic carbs, although the presence of fat causes less insulin to be released and a lower glycemic response, insulin is still present, which tells the body to store the calories as adipose tissue (fat).

That is why it is not such an exaggeration to say that a slice of pecan pie goes right to your waistline! But adding fat to a nutritious lower glycemic carbohydrate like sweet potatoes is a good idea because it will reduce the glycemic response even further and support the absorption of the fat-soluble vitamins too. Although eating carbs with fats will help to level out blood sugar and insulin spikes, it does not get rid of the insulin spike entirely. Remember that when insulin is present, fat storage increases. Therefore, limiting high glycemic and empty carbs overall is ideal.

HORMONE HIGHLIGHT: LEPTIN AND ADIPONECTIN

Our adipose tissue is responsible for manufacturing some very important metabolism-regulating hormones which play a key role in managing our hunger and stimulating fat burning:

- **Leptin** is secreted by fat cells after a meal when the body has received enough food/energy. When working correctly, elevated leptin levels signal our brain that we are satiated and tell us to stop eating. However, in people with **leptin resistance**, it is as if the brain is not getting those signals. Like an unresponsive teenager who tunes his mother out when she is knocking on his door to tell him it is time to do homework, the cells can no longer "hear" the leptin knocking on the cell walls to get in. So like the mom who keeps yelling while the teenager continues spacing out, the leptin levels might be elevated, but the receptors are not listening. Leptin resistance leads to hunger despite ingesting sufficient amounts of food, which can lead to uncontrolled eating, snacking, and even food obsessions and addiction. People with leptin resistance might have just eaten a meal but feel compelled to grab a burger and fries on their way home. Often, those with leptin resistance will carry a lot of guilt around food, because they have no control of their hunger urges. Leptin resistance can lead to a myriad of other problems because leptin is involved in regulating and signaling other important hormones: thyroid, adrenal, pancreatic, testosterone, and estrogen. In his book *Mastering Leptin*, Byron Richards, CCN, calls leptin "the most powerful hormone in the human body." Studies show that leptin resistance is also associated with elevated cholesterol.

❧ **Leptin and insulin.** Leptin works in tandem with insulin, which is released to bring down blood sugar levels when sugar and carbs are eaten. As we know, insulin resistance is when the body no longer recognizes insulin anymore, which can lead to prediabetes and eventually diabetes. The two hormones often spin out of balance together. When there is insulin or leptin resistance, it is very difficult to lose weight, and the body very easily gains weight. In this situation, calorie-counting is totally irrelevant. It all comes down to the type of calories we eat and our hormones. If you are leptin resistant, then your brain is not getting the signal that you are full, so you tend to overeat. Add in insulin resistance, and the body is also not going to recognize and process those calories in an efficient manner. This is a double-whammy to the metabolism. What causes leptin and insulin resistance? Eating too many processed and fast foods, the wrong fats (especially damaged and trans fats), inactivity, high levels of stress, foods with chemicals, and snacking all day long and into the evening. One of the keys to reversing leptin and insulin resistance is getting the right kind of exercise (see chapter ten), and using the Rule of Three for eating: each time you eat get your healthy fat, fiber, or protein.

❧ **Adiponectin.** Sometimes referred to as a "fat-burning hormone," adiponectin supports the body's processing of glucose and fats. Low levels of adiponectin have been associated with insulin resistance, increased inflammation, and a higher risk of coronary artery disease. Even though adiponectin is actually synthesized in the fat cells, having more fat cells does not mean that there will be more adiponectin. In fact, studies have found the opposite to be true. How can we boost our adiponectin levels to burn more fat? According to *Mastering Leptin* author Byron Richards, there are several ways: exercising, eating a high-fiber diet, eating antioxidant-rich fruits and vegetables, and consuming monounsaturated and high-quality omega-3 fatty acids. But perhaps the most important way to boost adiponectin levels is by upping our intake of one nutrient that approximately 70 percent of the population is estimated to be deficient in—magnesium! Foods rich in magnesium include dark leafy greens, nuts and seeds, legumes, and quinoa. But the best food source is raw cacao—the main ingredient in dark chocolate! Read more about magnesium and raw cacao in chapter eight, and turn to chapter sixteen for some delicious ways to incorporate raw cacao into your diet.

What about Cholesterol?

Cholesterol is a sterol, a kind of cousin to saturated fat. A very important hormone to our metabolism and overall health, cholesterol is needed for all of our cell membranes, to create bile acids, to synthesize vitamin D, and to manufacture other hormones.

Like saturated fats, cholesterol has been vilified as a contributor to heart disease. But new information is revealing that there isn't even a correlation between cholesterol and heart attacks. One study that looked at 130,000 people found nearly three-quarters of patients hospitalized for a heart attack actually had what were considered to be normal LDL cholesterol levels. A study published in the *Journal Clinical Nutrition* showed that in the aging population (over eighty-one), higher cholesterol levels are protective and linked to lower death rates. Another study published in the *Oxford Journal of Medicine and Health* concluded that higher levels of cholesterol may offer protection against infection and atherosclerosis. A 2008 Mt. Sinai School of Medicine study found that higher cholesterol levels in the elderly also equated to higher memory scores. According to *Grain Brain* author Dr. Perlmutter, "cholesterol is vitally important for brain function." He says that the recent changes in statin recommendations that could double prescriptions "present a worrisome proposition for brain health."

Dr. Mark Houston, author of *What Your Doctor May Not Tell You About Heart Disease*, says that "elevated cholesterol is not a sure sign of heart disease—any more than low levels are a promise of heart health." Dr. Houston says that heart disease begins with endothelium damage or dysfunction and then progresses through seven different "pathways": inflammation, oxidative stress, vascular autoimmunity, dyslipidemia, elevated blood pressure/blood sugar, and obesity. According to Dr. Houston, it is the oxidized (damaged) cholesterol that is damaging to the heart. What causes cholesterol to become oxidized? When the fats/cholesterol get damaged. One way this can happen is using damaged fats, or cooking foods with cholesterol at too high a heat. That is why runny sunny-side up eggs are better than hard-boiled and why cooking at a low and slow temperature is better than charbroiling. One way to avoid damaged cholesterol when grilling is to cook at a lower temperature and marinate your meats, which can protect the meat from free radical damage and oxidation. Buying organic or free range is also important when choosing foods that contain fat and cholesterol.

Are We Starving Our Brains and Damaging Our Nervous Systems?

Could our "healthy" low-fat diet literally have been starving our brain? Not only have we seen an increase in heart disease, cancer, and diabetes since the low-fat craze, we have also seen an exponential jump in cases of Alzheimer's, dementia, ADHD, depression, and other neurological issues. There is even a link between fatty acid deficiencies and violence. Our brain is largely fat. So eating a low-fat diet is kind of like putting your brain on a diet. And we certainly do not want to starve our brains! Without the right balance of fatty acids, many of which must be obtained from our food or supplements, the structure and functioning of the brain may be compromised.

Fat-Soluble Vitamins Need Fat!

Another problem with a diet that does not have enough fats is that we might end up with nutrient deficiencies. In order for our bodies to absorb fat-soluble vitamins (calcium, A, D, K, and E), they need fat molecules as "carriers." So even if you are eating lots of dark leafy greens, which are excellent sources of fat-soluble vitamins, unless you are having a little fat with them, you might not be absorbing all those nutrients. Drinking those fresh-pressed green juices? You might just as well be pouring some of that $10-a-bottle juice down the drain unless you are getting a little bit of fat with them (such as a handful of nuts or a couple teaspoons of chia seeds)! Fat-soluble vitamins are important for immunity, bone health, hormone regulation, and more. Vitamin A is associated with eye health and antiaging, vitamin K is responsible for healthy clotting, and vitamin E is important for sweeping free radicals.

Quick Overview of Fats

Healthy Fats (Enjoy)

High heat:

- Avocado oil. Avocado oil is great for salad dressings and can also be used as a cooking oil.

- Organic ghee (clarified butter). The lactose has been removed, so although it is a dairy product, it is not likely to bother those who can't handle lactose. In fact, ghee is wonderful for the digestion and has a very rich buttery taste.

Medium-high heat:

- Coconut oil. Look for the cold-pressed virgin variety. See more information on my favorite fat/oil of all below.

- Organic/grass-fed butter. (*Replace with ghee during dairy elimination.*) Contains CLA, which is a fat-burner.

- Virgin red palm oil. This oil is high in beta-carotenes.

- Organic lard or tallow. A traditional fat and a healthy option. I know—full circle, right?

Low-medium heat (all of the above, plus):

- ❧ Olive oil
- ❧ Fatty fish

Raw/no heat (all of the above, plus):

- ❧ Fish oils
- ❧ Chia seeds/flaxseeds/hemp seeds
- ❧ Nut oils

For more information on fish and nut oils and chia, flax, and hemp seeds, see chapter six on inflammation.

Unhealthy Fats (Avoid)

- ❧ Trans fats (partially hydrogenated oils). This includes margarines.
- ❧ Spray "butters" or butter spreads. These often contain a chemical that provides a "butter flavor" which is potentially carcinogenic.
- ❧ Canola (rapeseed) oil
- ❧ Vegetable oils
- ❧ Cottonseed oil
- ❧ Soy oil. This is a sneaky one. It may not be something you pick up in the oil and vinegar section of the store, but it is found in most bottled dressings, mayonnaise, sports and cereal bars, and many packaged and processed foods. So if you are eating a lot of prepared and processed foods, you are getting a lot of soy in your diet even though you did not know it.

My Favorite Fats (Use Liberally!)

1. Coconut Oil—The Perfect Fat

If you had told me a few years ago that I would be taking coconut oil by the spoonful and putting it into tea, coffee, and smoothies, I would have said you were crazy, loco, mad! I mean, who in their right mind would purposely sit down and eat saturated fat by the spoonful? But that is exactly what I am doing! I have found coconut oil to be one of the critical pieces to the metabolism puzzle—almost magical really. In Sanskrit, coconuts are called *kalpa vriksha* which means: "The tree that gives all that is necessary for life." It is a well-earned name because coconut oil is pretty much the perfect fat with unique health and metabolism benefits. Let's take a look at some of coconut oil's unique benefits:

- It boosts our energy and stimulates the metabolism. Coconut oil is a medium chain fatty acid, which gets converted to energy and is burned as fuel faster (so it is less likely to be stored as fat). A Brazilian study found that consuming two tablespoons of coconut oil daily was linked to a reduction in belly fat and improved cholesterol markers.

- It is beneficial for the heart. Coconut oil contains about 50 percent lauric acid, which helps in preventing various heart problems including high cholesterol levels and high blood pressure. Coconut oil boosts HDL cholesterol, which is the good cholesterol that helps to usher out bad cholesterol.

- The polyphenols and lauric acid it contains boost the immune system, and its caprylic acid helps to fight fungal, bacterial, and viral infections.

- It helps to keep blood sugar level and reduces cravings.

- Like other fats, coconut oil improves our body's ability to absorb important fat-soluble vitamins and minerals such as calcium, magnesium, and vitamins K and D, which are necessary for the development of strong bones.

- Coconut oil has also been shown to help boost and balance the thyroid gland.

- Its natural antiviral and antibacterial properties mean that coconut oil can support digestion and cleansing; it can even be used as a natural deodorant (internal and external)!

- Because of its natural antibacterial qualities, coconut oil helps to remove bacteria from the mouth and supports detox/cleansing. Called "oil-pulling," you simply swish a tablespoon of virgin coconut oil around in the mouth for about ten minutes, then spit it out (don't swallow it because there will be bacteria in it).

- Coconut oil is moisturizing as well as being antibacterial/viral, which makes it ideal topically for various skin problems including psoriasis, dermatitis, eczema, or skin infections.

- Coconut oil is also touted to boost brain functioning (potentially even lowering the risk of or reducing the symptoms of Alzheimer's). Some experts recommend taking three to four tablespoons a day for Alzheimer's or dementia prevention.

How to Get Your Coconut Oil

There are a number of ways to consume coconut oil. I recommend starting with one to three teaspoons daily. You may gradually work up to three tablespoons if you desire:

- Sauté your veggies in it. Your body absorbs fat-soluble vitamins better when they are consumed with a healthy fat like coconut oil. Some people even like to take their multivitamin with a little coconut oil to improve absorption of the fat soluble vitamins.

- Make homemade dark chocolates (see recipes).

- Put a spoonful of coconut oil into your coffee or tea. I have found this to be helpful if I am craving sugar; it can help to "turn off" those cravings.

- Scoop out and eat coconut flesh.

- Eat coconut butter, drink coconut milk, or add it to smoothies/recipes.

Want more ideas and recipes for coconut oil? Read *The Coconut Oil Miracle* by Bruce Fife or *Eat Fat, Lose Fat* by Dr. Mary Enig and Sally Fallon.

2. Chia Seeds

Chia seeds are the reason I became a nutritionist, because when I started to eat them every day, I could not believe the amazing impact they had on my energy, digestion, endurance, mood, and overall health. An ancient Aztec superfood, chia seeds gave their warriors the long-lasting energy, focus, and endurance needed to go into battle. An excellent source of inflammation-lowering omega-3 fatty acids, chia seeds are also high in protein and contain a number of minerals including calcium, magnesium, and potassium. Omega-3s are proven brain and mood food and reduce the risk of many diseases from breast cancer to heart disease. Unlike flaxseed, which is also a good source of vegan omega-3s, chia seeds are rich in antioxidants, which makes them more stable, keeps them from going rancid after grinding, and helps to prevent free radical damage.

Chia seeds are uniquely *hydrophilic*, meaning that when the seed comes in contact with water, it soaks up about ten times its own weight forming a gel-like substance. Chia gel helps to fill us up, slows the absorption of sugar into the bloodstream, levels out blood sugar, sweeps toxins out of the body, and maintains hydration. Because of this, it is important to always make sure to consume chia seeds with plenty of water or liquids to prevent them from soaking up moisture inside your digestive tract—which could dehydrate you! Soak chia seeds for about five minutes before consuming to ensure they are well-hydrated. Some people need time to adjust to the fiber, so start with a teaspoon of well-hydrated chia seeds first.

3. Avocado

Another healthy fat that I absolutely love is avocado. Avocados help to reduce our inflammation, boost the absorption of certain fat-soluble vitamins, and are a good source of carotenoids, folate, potassium, and vitamins K, B5, B6, and C. Avocados promote bone and heart health and help manage blood sugar. Adding avocados to smoothies can make them light and fluffy, boost the fiber and vitamin content, and keep you satisfied longer. Avocados are also an excellent source of fiber, which like chia seeds, makes them somewhat unique among fats. One of my favorite things to teach kids is to "eat an avocado a day to keep the doctor away!"

How Much Fat Should We Eat?

So how much fat is it healthy to have in our diets? The answer is it depends. You need to eat enough that you are not craving sugar and simple carbs. Swapping out a serving or two of carbs for a food that is rich in high-quality fats is a good start. On average, it appears that most people will benefit from about 40 percent of total caloric intake coming from healthy fats, but some experts contend that people will benefit from even higher levels!

GALLBLADDER ISSUES?

Do You Have Trouble Digesting Fats?

If you have gallbladder issues, you might be cringing as you are reading this chapter because the idea of eating more fats might sound like a nightmare. When your gallbladder is not working well, you can have more trouble processing fats.

The gallbladder sits below the liver and stores and concentrates bile from the liver, which is used to break down and digest fats. Most fats (except coconut oil) require bile salts for digestion. Bile also assists in the proper absorption of your fat-soluble vitamins (A, D, E, and K).

So if you are one of the 25 million Americans with gallbladder issues, you might sometimes have trouble eating fatty foods. This could make the idea of increasing your fat intake unpleasant or even downright impossible.

Why are gallbladder problems at such epidemic proportions in this country? In addition to heredity, age, and gender (women are more likely to suffer), here are some more possible reasons:

- Diets too high in processed foods/bad fats (such as trans fats and oxidized oils found in margarines and packaged foods)

- Diets too high in sugar

- Yo-yo dieting/extreme weight loss

- Not enough healthy fats (Paradoxically low-fat diets stress the gallbladder, which makes fats difficult to digest, which causes reduced-fat intake, and more stress on gallbladder.)

- Vitamin B6 depletion (caused by stress, birth control pills, hormone replacement therapy)—*this is a BIG one for gallbladder health!*

- Food intolerances (Eggs are a common gallbladder foe.)

- Other risk factors including obesity, diabetes, ethnicity

- Low HDL cholesterol (which ushers the bad cholesterol out of the body)

The symptoms of gallbladder issues include gas, bloating, reflux, pain in the right side (might radiate up) after meals—especially fatty ones—and poor absorption of fats. You can often tell if you are not absorbing and digesting fats if you have light, loose, or floating stools (yes, you should look before you flush!). Also, scaly, dry, cracking, or bumpy "chicken" skin—often seen on the back of the arms or with cracking heels—can be another indicator that your diet is deficient in fatty acids. If your diet is deficient in fats, then you will likely also have deficiencies in fat-soluble vitamins.

If you do have gallbladder trouble, you will likely want to take this program more slowly and increase the fats more gradually, emphasize one specific fat—coconut oil. Unlike other fats, coconut oil does not require bile salts for digestion. For that reason, it tends to be better tolerated and digested more easily than other fats.

How to Prime Your Gallbladder for Eating Fats!

To support fat digestion, try this digestive tonic before your meal:

Mix the following into four to six ounces of water, and drink it right before your meals:

- 1 teaspoon of Bragg apple cider vinegar (must use raw apple cider vinegar with the "mother")
- Juice from half of a lemon
- A dash or pinch of pink Himalayan salt

You could also carry digestive enzymes with you; make sure to find one that has a broad range of enzymes including lipase and/or ox bile to support the digestion of fats. Bitters can also help. Taking a high-quality multivitamin with the full B complex (including B6) supports the gallbladder.

Please note: If you have had your gallbladder removed or are having issues with it, please consult with your doctor before embarking on this program.

The Bottom Line

Back in 2002, Gary Taubes wrote a groundbreaking article published in the *New York Times* called "What If It's All Been a Big Fat Lie?" which exposed the low and no-fat craze as disastrous for our health. Finally, over a decade later, we are starting to see the tides change. But unfortunately, millions of Americans have suffered the consequences of the low-fat craze. It is time to put the idea to rest for good that low-fat foods are better for our weight and health.

Once you start including healthy fats into your diet, you will be able to gain more control of your hunger, blood sugar, and moods. Many people notice that their skin appears smoother and less wrinkled too. The critical point here is that the *quality* of the fat matters. If you choose butter or beef, it should be from a grass-fed cow. Avoid damaged fats. When you are craving sugar or carbs, reach for a handful of nuts, a half an avocado, or a cup of tea with a spoonful of coconut oil in it instead. You should see your skin improve, your hunger decrease, and your cells will thank you. This is what a perfect metabolism is all about.

❧ 3 ❧

Heal the Gut
Balance Digestion and the Inner Ecosystem

New science indicates that damage to your digestive tract heads the list of priorities for debugging stubborn weight issues. This is likely true whether you think you have digestive problems or not.

—BYRON RICHARDS, CCN

It is estimated that 70 million Americans suffer from digestive issues. Often, people have lived with digestive issues for so long that they just think of them as normal or feel as though there is nothing they can do to fix them. They may not even mention them to their doctor or nutritionist! Others have sought treatment or even had surgery, yet continue to suffer. A healthy digestive system is the foundation to good health, and gut imbalances could offer clues to many of our confounding health problems.

Some of the symptoms of digestive trouble can include:

- ❧ chronic constipation
- ❧ frequent heartburn or reflux
- ❧ bloating, gas, or pain after meals
- ❧ floating, light-colored, loose, or very foul-smelling stools
- ❧ diarrhea, loss of bowel control
- ❧ a feeling of fullness in the bowel

According to Hippocrates, the father of modern medicine, "all disease begins in the gut." The ancient tradition of Ayurvedic medicine also believes that optimal health can only be achieved if digestive problems are resolved.

Gut health imbalances can obviously cause digestive disorders. But because our gut is the foundation of our overall immune systems and health, imbalances can also generate many other seemingly unrelated chronic health problems ranging from unexplained aches and pains to neurological issues, mood disorders, chronic inflammation, diseases, and a sluggish metabolism/stubborn weight gain.

Why Is Digestion Important?

Our digestive system plays many roles and serves many purposes in the body:

1. **Delivers nutrients.** What we eat cannot provide nourishment or energy until it has been broken down into particles that can be delivered, absorbed, and utilized by the body. Our digestive system is kind of like the Amazon.com of our body—it packages up the things that we eat so they can be delivered to the cells. If our digestive system has a breakdown, our food just does not get properly processed, so the cells get starved and the inventory just starts to pile up.

2. **Provides a barrier.** Our intestines form a barricade designed to let in nutrients while keeping out toxic substances. It is kind of like a bouncer at a high-end nightclub who is paid to make sure that the people entering the club are not going to cause trouble. The bouncer eyeballs everyone and decides who to let in and who to keep out. If the junctions in our barrier wall get damaged, they can become "leaky" and let some toxins and partially digested proteins into the bloodstream—like a bouncer who is allowing troublemakers to sneak by. The immune system then revs up to attack the leaked toxins. A leaky gut is linked to many health issues including bloating, asthma, eczema, skin conditions, food sensitivities, fibromyalgia, joint pain, irritable bowel syndrome, other digestive disorders, and even diabetes, autoimmune conditions, and hypothyroidism.

3. **Removes toxins and waste.** Our digestive system also needs to effectively remove toxins and waste products from the body. In this sense, it operates like waste management: If the garbage trucks go on strike for a few weeks, all that refuse can quickly

pile up and start to stink. Similarly, our digestive system needs to be effectively and very regularly removing the waste matter, or it can accumulate. *See chapter five on toxins to learn more about this aspect of digestion.*

If there is a breakdown in any of the many stages of digestion, the body could become undernourished, vulnerable to chemicals and infections, overburdened with toxins, or any combination of the three. Let's take a step back and look at how the system is supposed to operate.

How Does Digestion Work?

Our digestion begins before we even take a bite of food. The smell, sight, and anticipation of food cause us to salivate as a first stage. Saliva contains amylase, a digestive enzyme that helps break down starches (polysaccharides). Our teeth masticate or tear our food into smaller pieces. Those particles mix with the saliva, which moisten them and helps to bind them together to create what is called a bolus. A bolus can easily travel down through our esophagus and into our stomach. For this stage of digestion, it is important to slow down and thoroughly chew our food.

After food leaves our mouth, it travels through the esophagus using peristaltic contractions to get down to our stomach. In the stomach, our gastric acids and more digestive enzymes break the food down into particles that can be absorbed and used by the body. Referred to as our "digestive fire," our natural gastric acid and digestive enzymes are needed to properly process what we eat. But our body's supply of enzymes naturally declines as we age. Certain medications (such as antihistamines, proton pump inhibitors, and antacids), and highly processed diets can also lower our natural production of hydrochloric acid and digestive enzymes. Without a sufficient "digestive fire," the amino acids and nutrients we take in may not be fully assimilated from our foods. This can cause problems like indigestion, constipation, gas, and discomfort. Our gastric acids also make our gut inhospitable to microorganisms and bacteria. Having an insufficient digestive fire can be an invitation for bacteria and infections to set up shop.

Why We Get Hooked on Antacids

Reflux and indigestion are very common problems for people eating a Western diet. Although it might seem that indigestion is caused by excess stomach acid, more often than not it happens *because there is not enough*. When our stomach acid is low, we do not have what we need to properly break down and digest our foods. This low acid state paradoxically causes the partially digested food particles (and the acid that is there) to come back up. Heartburn can be extremely painful and can even lead to serious diseases. So it is no surprise that people turn to acid blockers to get relief. But although antacids and proton pump inhibitors (PPIs) can relieve symptoms, they work against digestion by neutralizing gastric juices—exactly the opposite of what most people need. That is how we get hooked: because they further reduce our stomach acid, taking them works against digestion in the long term. So what can people with reflux and indigestion do? For starters, eat fewer processed foods and more raw, living foods with enzymes (but take it slow, gradually adding in more fiber and enzyme-rich foods to avoid gas and bloating). Other very important things are taking a daily probiotic and/or digestive enzymes before meals and identifying and removing foods that tend to trigger attacks (alcohol, spicy foods, chocolate, eggs). Reflux is also a very common symptom of food sensitivities. Because reflux can progress to a very dangerous condition, I recommend trying a food elimination diet or having a food intolerance panel run to diagnose any sensitivities (*see the next chapter for more information about this*). A supplement called zinc-carnosine may also be helpful for reflux sufferers.

Your Second Brain

Whenever someone tells me they have anxiety, my next question is always, "How is your digestion?" Why? Because the gut is our "second brain."

We all are familiar with the brain in our skulls hard at work whether we are taking notes in a philosophy class, trying to balance our checkbook, or doing a Words with Friends puzzle. But we all are equipped with another brain inside our gut. First called "the second brain" by Dr. Michael Gershon, our gut is lined with a complex and extensive set of neurons called the enteric nervous system. The expressions "gut reaction" or "follow your gut" help to explain what our second brain does— guide our feelings, moods, certain behaviors, and reactions. If we touch a hot pot on the stove, it is our second brain that tells us to pull back quickly. If we waited for our cerebral brain to ponder the positives and negatives of keeping our hand on the pot, it would surely get burned. The gut is also responsible for manufacturing important neurotransmitters that play a role in our mood and brain function—one of which is serotonin, often referred to as "the happiness hormone." Over 95 percent of our serotonin is found in our gut, so it makes absolute sense that our moods are tied to the health of our digestive system and explains why having digestive trouble for a long period of time can lead to brain chemistry imbalances that can drive depression, anxiety, mood disorders, and ADHD. A 2013 Swedish study found a link between functional abdominal pain and feelings of anxiety and depression, even in those with mild gastrointestinal symptoms. And when our neurotransmitters are out of balance, it can lead to cravings and addictions.

The Role of Bacteria

Bacteria play an extremely important role in our metabolism and digestive and immune system health. Perhaps their role is bigger than we currently realize. Humans have trillions of bacteria in our bodies; in fact we are made up of ten times more bacterial cells than human cells, so technically we are more bacterial than human! Bacteria live in our digestive system, our skin, and mucous membranes—our bodies are literally teeming with them. There are between 500 and 1,000 different types of bacteria in our guts alone!

When it comes to bacteria, it is all about balance. Alongside the "good guys" in our digestive system, it is normal to have some "bad guys" or disease-causing bacteria like E. coli, candida, and salmonella. As long as we have enough friendly bacteria to keep the disease-causing microorganisms in check, they cannot grow out of control and cause issues with our digestion, immunity, and overall health. Research shows that ideally we should have twenty times more beneficial bacteria than the unhealthy kind to maintain a healthy immune and digestive system. You want to "stack your team" and guarantee a win in every match. A balanced inner ecosystem is very important for digestion, immunity, mood, and even has an impact on your weight. There is some very good research suggesting that this could be a factor in the fight against heart disease and diabetes. But there are a number of things strengthening the opposing team, one of which is the rampant overuse of antibiotics.

Antibiotics and Antibacterials Are Backfiring

In 1928, Sir Alexander Fleming first discovered a mold that could kill bacteria. He called it penicillin. It was put into use in the 1940s, and the results were miraculous! Bacterial infections that had been slowly and painfully killing people could now be cured. But since then, antibiotics have been grossly overprescribed. Because of this, bacteria have been evolving, and new resistant strains have developed. An increasing number of people are now carriers of staph bacteria, and we are seeing a giant spike in the incidence of MRSA infections, especially among teenagers. Some experts are predicting an end to the antibiotic era is nearing.

The thing is, antibiotic and antibacterial agents wipe out bacteria, but take down the "good guys" along with the bad guys. And it is very important for the good to outnumber the bad. The overuse of antibiotics and antibacterial agents (like triclosan) is creating problems ranging from resistant bacteria to weight gain. Some studies also show that antibacterial agents not only inhibit bacteria, but they could also be inhibiting hormones.

More than 80 percent of the antibiotics used in the United States will be fed to livestock. Animals raised in factory farms are regularly given low "subtherapeutic" doses of antibiotics to prevent and reverse diseases passed between animals living in close quarters and to fatten them up. But this continual supply of antibiotics is creating resistant strains of bacteria in our meat supply. *Read more about this in chapter four.*

Fight the Good Fight—with Bacteria

According to a Cherokee legend, a grandfather sits down with his grandson to tell him the story of the two wolves. He says,

> *"Grandson, there is a fight going on inside of you every day. It is a terrible battle between two wolves. One wolf is evil—he is anger, pain, greed, sorrow, ego, guilt, arrogance, false pride, disease, hatred, and mistrust. The other wolf is empathy, generosity, kindness, faith, serenity, hope, humility, love, health, joy, and compassion. This very same fight is happening inside of me, and inside of every human being." The grandson ponders this for a moment,*

then asks, "Well, which wolf wins?" The grandfather pauses before responding, "Whichever one you feed."

This is exactly what is going on inside each and every one of our guts every day.

Beyond Our Gut

Because 70 percent of our immune system resides in our gut, this region of the body is the foundation of our overall immune system and health. When our digestive system is not in good shape, it can set up a cascade of problems ranging from frequent viruses and infections to chronic inflammation and related diseases. Studies show that probiotics can be a powerful tool in boosting the body's immune response to fight off certain infectious agents and inflammatory conditions.

What probiotics do is shore up the good bacteria in the digestive system that help ward off and treat many gastrointestinal disorders including IBS, constipation, diarrhea, inflammatory bowel disease, and reflux. Statistics show that nearly 65 million people are regularly constipated. Bowels that are congested (that's what constipation is) store toxins that can accumulate in the large intestine. This can lead to illness, low energy, and discomfort. Probiotics are a key component in resolving this condition. They might even help to combat bad breath, fibromyalgia, and diabetes.

Could Probiotics Be the New Weight Loss Pills?

Studies show that there is a powerful connection between our weight and the type of bacteria in our gut. According to the *New York Times*, "the bacterial makeup of the intestines may help determine whether people gain weight or lose it, according to two new studies." These studies found that as much as 20 percent of the weight loss from gastric bypass surgery might actually be attributed to a shift in gut bacteria. The reason could be that bacteria are closely tied to our hormones like insulin and leptin, which affect our body's ability to process sugars, regulate appetite, and our energy. So before taking such drastic measures as gastric bypass surgery to lose weight, perhaps turning to probiotics and fermented foods and drinks will be the new magic "weight loss pills."

Gut Bacteria Is Linked to Heart Disease

A recent study conducted at the Cleveland Clinic demonstrated a link between heart disease and gut bacteria. The researchers found that foods containing lecithin, carnitine, and choline can interact with certain intestinal bacteria during metabolism to increase the risk of heart attacks by releasing a substance converted by the liver to a chemical known as TMAO (trimethylamine N-oxide). Elevated blood levels of TMAO are linked to increased risk of stroke and heart attack. In both studies, when the subjects were given antibiotics, the risk went away. But as soon as the antibiotics were stopped, the risk returned. Since taking antibiotics continually is not an acceptable option, what is left is avoidance of the particular trigger foods (includes eggs and meat), or perhaps better—changing gut bacteria by taking a probiotic to balance the bacterial load in the intestines to prevent the reaction.

Fermented Foods

Fermentation has been used for centuries as a method of preserving foods before refrigeration. Not only does it prevent food from spoiling, fermentation keeps the minerals and vitamins alive, and can even manufacture new ones (like vitamin K and the B vitamins)! Additionally, foods that have been fermented contain beneficial bacteria (probiotics) and enzymes to improve our digestion, boost our immune systems, and provide energy. Fermentation basically turns regular foods into superfoods! Fermented foods are a delicious way to get healthy bacteria into the gut. Possibilities include kimchi, traditional sauerkraut and fermented pickles, kombucha, kefir, yogurt, buttermilk, miso (fermented soybean paste), traditional sourdough (which could be why some people who do not digest wheat bread well, can handle it), and raw apple cider vinegar. Many cultures around the world have their own traditional fermented food; the Korean Food Research Institute estimates that the average adult Korean eats more than a quarter pound of kimchi daily!

How Do You Know If Your Digestion Is Working Well?

You should not be constipated. You should have a well-formed, firm, but not dry bowel movement *every single day*. Yes, every day. It is *very* important to keep the bowels moving. See below for some tips for dealing with constipation.

You should not have bloating, discomfort, diarrhea, or reflux after you eat or anytime during the day or night. Bloating and discomfort can signal a food intolerance. If you are experiencing any kind of bloating or reflux, keep a diary of when this happens and determine what you ate before an onset. Such symptoms could also be from low stomach acid, a bacterial/candida overgrowth, or a gut infection.

You should get energy from your food not feel sluggish and tired after eating. If you are feeling sluggish after a meal, you could be lacking in the enzymes and stomach juices needed to properly digest the food. You might have a food intolerance as well. There could be candida or an overgrowth of yeast bacteria or adrenal fatigue. You could also have some nutritional deficiencies, especially within the B vitamins.

You should not have loose or floating stools. Floating stools could indicate a problem absorbing fats, which can result from a leaky gut, food intolerance, parasite, or infection. It can also be an indication of liver congestion and gallbladder trouble. Having more than six bowel movements daily can also be an indication of digestive trouble.

Nine Tips to Support Digestion

1. **Sit down.** Multitasking is not good for the digestion. When we eat, we should be focused on the task of eating. Be seated at the table when you eat, avoid eating on the run or in front of the television or computer. This establishes more mindfulness around food and supports digestion.

2. **Slow down.** Before you even begin to eat, pause and look at your food, which causes the salivary glands to begin working for the first stage of digestion. Then chew each bite of your food thoroughly. Ayurveda views chewing as very important to the digestive process. Many people do not eat slowly enough or chew their food properly. Traditional Ayurveda says that each bite should be chewed thirty-two times—even if we all made it to half that number, it would be an improvement.

3. **Calm down.** Avoid arguing when you eat, as elevated stress releases hormones that interfere with digestion. Avoid trying to solve your problems and issues while eating; this can interfere with digestion too.

4. **Boost.** Certain foods are very supportive to our digestion:

   a. High-fiber foods like chia seeds (when properly hydrated) help to boost motility and keep us "regular."

   b. Fresh ginger can be soothing to the stomach.

   c. Fermented foods provide healthy bacteria and easily absorbable nutrients which can be very helpful in boosting digestion.

   d. Having a glass of lemon water mixed with a teaspoon of raw apple cider vinegar shortly before a meal can also help to boost digestion.

5. **Hydrate.** We need to drink plenty of water each day for proper hydration, cellular function, and to support efficient

elimination. Many Americans are chronically dehydrated. Even mild dehydration can lead to constipation, decrease our athletic performance, cause the body to hold on to toxins, and even raise our risk of a heart event. Relying on thirst may not be a good guide because when we are chronically dehydrated, our thirst mechanism may not be working optimally. Read chapter nine for more information about hydration.

6. **Don't dilute.** Drinking too much water with your food can reduce your digestive enzymes/fire. Especially avoid drinking alkaline water with a meal, which can neutralize the acid in the stomach and interfere with digestion.

7. **Eliminate.** If there is an infection present, it will be next to impossible to heal the gut. Identifying and eradicating bacterial imbalances, infections, parasites, or food intolerances will be critical. If you suspect an infection or food intolerance, check with your health practitioner about obtaining a stool test that can diagnose infections of parasites and/or having a food intolerance test run. Having a sluggish thyroid can also lead to chronic constipation, so testing thyroid levels is also a good idea.

8. **Detox.** If our digestion is overburdened with toxins and chemicals, that can slow things down. It is a good idea to give the digestion a much-needed break a couple of times a year with a supportive detox protocol.

9. **Support.** There are a number of ways to support healthy digestion:

    a. Digestive enzymes taken at the beginning of a meal can assist in the absorption and digestion of foods and be very helpful for people who are lacking enzymes or suffer digestive trouble.

    b. Aloe vera juice (inner fillet) can be a lifesaver for those with constipation or a sluggish/sensitive digestive system. Take one to two tablespoons daily before bedtime.

    c. Chia seeds soak up about ten times their own weight in water, which creates a gel that supports healthy elimination and helps to draw toxins. If you are not used to fiber in your diet, work up gradually from one teaspoon to two or three tablespoons daily. Allow the seeds to soak in plenty of liquid for five minutes first.

d. Zinc-carnosine has been shown in several studies to be helpful for some reflux and ulcer sufferers.

e. Triphala fruit is an Ayurvedic herbal formula that enhances healthy digestion and bowel movements. It also has been recognized to support the liver and blood cleansing.

f. Probiotics boost the good bacteria and crowd out the bad ones. These are found in fermented foods or drinks or a high-quality probiotic supplement. Adding a prebiotic fiber can further help to feed the probiotics and support colonization of good bacteria, but note that prebiotics can lead to gas in some people, especially those with IBS.

g. L-glutamine is helpful in repairing and rebuilding damage to the gut lining (but it can be constipating, so avoid if you are not regular).

h. Magnesium can relax the bowel and prevent constipation. Avoid the oxide form because it is poorly absorbed. I prefer the malate, orotate, citrate, or glycinate forms. You can also use a magnesium spray or get magnesium by soaking in an Epsom or sea salt bath (one cup of salts in bathwater, soak no longer than twenty minutes, rinse off in shower). *Those with an existing medical condition such as diabetes should consult their doctor first.*

I certainly suffered from my fair share of digestion problems. I was plagued by chronic constipation for more than half of my life. And unfortunately, like many Americans, I thought that was just "normal" for me, so I suffered along. My digestion can still become sluggish when I travel, get a little dehydrated, or find myself out of my routine or eating foods that don't support my digestion. But the thing is, because I have experienced a healthy digestive system, one day of constipation is unacceptable to me now—two days literally unbearable! I have absolutely no idea how I lived through three to five days of constipation on a regular basis as a child!

The Bottom Line

When our gut is unhealthy, many other areas of our metabolism and health suffer. Because 70 percent of our immune system resides in our gut, living with digestive troubles can be a recipe for disaster for our overall health. When our digestive system is not in good shape, it can set us up for a cascade of problems ranging from bloating and weight gain to frequent colds and infections, nutrient deficiencies, chronic inflammation, allergies, food sensitivities, mood imbalances like anxiety, and even diseases.

4

Identify Food Intolerances
Are Some Foods Making You Foggy, Fatigued, and Fat?

There is a voice that does not use words. Listen.   —RUMI

What Are Our Bodies Trying to Tell Us? Are We Listening?

Our bodies communicate with us all day long, not in words, but with symptoms. Headaches, fatigue, hunger, pain, fever—are all examples of the body trying to tell us something. But our instinct is to do everything we can to quiet our bodies down! This is like giving a pacifier to a fussing baby: sure, it might calm her down for a little while, but if the fuss is over hunger or a wet diaper, the pacifier just prolongs the discomfort. Instead of just treating our symptoms, we ideally want to determine what is causing them. That might be easier said than done if they are vague or come and go seemingly without reason.

What if the answers to many of your perplexing symptoms—including unexplained weight gain, foggy brain, migraines, rashes, chronic fatigue, and aches and pains—were right at the end of your fork? What if an intolerance to a common food that you eat every day has been responsible for your weight gain and a myriad of chronic and seemingly unrelated health problems?

If you are like most people, you might be tempted to skip to the next chapter right now because you are probably thinking: *"I don't have any food sensitivities, this doesn't apply to me."* Perhaps you are right, but please don't skip this chapter! Food intolerances can be very sneaky. I am here to tell you that *not knowing* could be hurting you. For every person who has identified a food intolerance, there are likely many more people living with undiagnosed ones.

Avoiding gluten and other foods might just seem like a passing trend, but there are many real problems associated with food intolerances. It is important to identify sensitivities because they are linked to a growing list of chronic and serious health issues including arthritis, heart disease, thyroid problems, autoimmune diseases, diabetes, and more.

Three Reasons You May Have Missed a Food Intolerance

1. **Food intolerances get confused with food allergies.** True food allergies, which can lead to life-threatening symptoms like swelling of the airway and low blood pressure, are relatively rare, affecting only about 4 percent of the population. On the other hand, food intolerances are likely very prevalent, affecting a much larger segment of the population. With a food allergy, the immune system recognizes the offending food as harmful and produces antibodies to fight it, causing an immunoglobulin E (IgE) reaction and the release of histamine. Even tiny amounts of the offending food can cause a reaction, which can affect the digestive system (vomiting, diarrhea), respiratory system (coughing, runny nose, asthma), and/or skin (itchiness, hives, rash).

   While food allergies can be tested for using a positive skin prick or blood test, food intolerance reactions can be vaguer and affect many other organs in the body including muscles, joints, the brain, the heart, and the thyroid. The symptoms and possible complications of food intolerances are extensive and can include:

   - Acne
   - Alopecia (hair loss)
   - Anxiety
   - Anemia
   - Arthritis and joint aches
   - Asthma
   - ADHD, hyperactivity, behavior issues
   - Autoimmune conditions

- Autism

- Bed-wetting

- Blood sugar issues

- Brain fog, forgetfulness, focus issues

- Dark circles under the eyes ("shiners")

- Digestive trouble such as gas, bloating, reflux, diarrhea, constipation, irritable bowel

- Fatigue and a general feeling of malaise

- Frequent colds and infections, lowered immunity

- Hormone issues such as PCOS or infertility

- Itchiness

- Insomnia

- Migraines, headaches

- Mood disorders such as depression, OCD, crying spells

- Mouth ulcers/canker sores

- Muscle and joint aches or fibromyalgia

- Numbness, tingling, or nerve problems

- Runny nose, sneezing

- Stunted growth in kids

- Sleep issues

- Skin conditions including eczema, rashes, acne, etc.

- Thyroid issues including Graves' and Hashimoto's

- Upper respiratory symptoms like sneezing fits, a runny nose, or chronic coughs

- Weight gain/weight loss

- Even diseases are being linked to food intolerances, including schizophrenia, heart disease, Alzheimer's, diabetes, and others

2. **Food intolerance reactions can be delayed.** Someone with a food allergy typically knows about it right away because the reaction occurs quickly. Even tiny amounts of the food can lead to a reaction. Some food intolerance reactions can be immediate, others can also be delayed. It can take sometimes up to

forty-eight hours for the substance to create a symptom, and again, the symptom may not be an obvious "reaction." This can make it seem next to impossible to connect the reaction to the particular food that caused it. Quite often, food intolerances develop from eating foods that we enjoy all the time, so that can make it even more complicated to link the food to the reaction.

3. **We learn to tune it out and shrug it off.** Our bodies, in their infinite wisdom, kind of learn to cope with chronic food sensitivities. Maybe a food reaction shows up as chronic knee pain or tennis elbow. It's so easy to explain them away: "I have knee trouble from pounding the pavement too much." "I have tennis elbow because I play four matches a week." But why then doesn't your running mate or tennis partner seem to have the same trouble? It comes down to the body's inflammatory response.

Food intolerances can create chronic inflammation in the body. Often because we are eating the offending foods all day long, we experience some chronic symptoms all of the time, and we simply do not connect the symptoms to the foods that we are eating.

I call this "The Grand Central Station Phenomenon."

Picture this. You are sitting on a bench in Grand Central Station during rush hour. You drop a single pin. Do you think you could hear that little pin hitting the floor among all the din? Probably not. There is too much going on around you to focus on that tiny little sound. In the same way, our bodies learn to tune out reactions to certain foods.

But if you drop the same pin while lying quietly in a peaceful room, you will probably hear it loud and clear. The principle behind a food elimination diet is similar: we remove certain foods to take away all the "noise," and then when we reintroduce them, we can really listen to what our bodies are trying to say.

Hypochondriac or Food Intolerance?

It is very common for someone to suffer with a long list of chronic and vague symptoms for years before even considering a food intolerance as the source. Sadly, many people will never link foods to their symptoms. I used to pacify my own chronic aches and pains with Advil until

I finally got relief by removing gluten from my diet a few years ago. Food intolerances can get someone labeled as a "hypochondriac" because they seem to never feel quite right or have a long and growing list of health complaints. As a child, I continually complained of a sore throat, itchy red eyes, constipation, and had allergic "shiners."

Elimination Diet/Challenge

One way to determine if your health issues or stubborn weight gain could be due to food intolerances is to try a food elimination diet and challenge. The way it works is that common "problem" foods are removed for a period of time, generally one to three weeks. Afterward they are brought back into the diet one by one (with at least twenty-four hours between) to see if there is a reaction. If there is a reaction, the offending food should be removed again for three to six months on average. After a longer period of avoidance, it can then be reintroduced again to see if there is a reaction.

Common Food Intolerances

The list of foods to which we can be intolerant is virtually endless, but a handful of foods are generally the top offenders. These include:

- Gluten, wheat, and gluten-containing grains
- Dairy products
- Genetically modified organisms (GMOs), especially corn and soy
- Eggs can be trouble for some but also contribute to a healthy metabolism in those who are not sensitive, so removing eggs is optional.

Let's take a closer look how each of these key foods can be wreaking havoc on your weight and health.

Whole Wheat/Gluten

Ten years ago, most people had not even heard of gluten. Today, it is estimated that almost a third of the population is avoiding gluten at least to some extent. But many still wonder whether it is a fad or if there is a real reason everyone from celebrities and famous athletes to your next-door neighbor seems to be jumping on the gluten-free bandwagon.

I am here to tell you that it is not a fad. The evidence is mounting that gluten and other food intolerances could be contributing to our weight gain and many other health problems. Giving up gluten and wheat can be life-changing for many people; it certainly was for me. A lot of the confusion around gluten is that many people assume that as long as you don't have celiac disease, you should be able to handle gluten just fine. But the truth is many serious and debilitating symptoms can be traced back to non-celiac gluten sensitivity.

But Isn't Whole Grain Healthy?

For years we have been told that whole wheat is better for us because it contains whole grains and fiber. Yes, fiber helps to level out blood sugar and support digestion, so common sense would tell us that whole wheat is better for us. But as we know from chapter one, a lot of whole wheat items are just processed foods made of enriched wheat flour. But that is not the whole story . . .

Dr. William Davis, author of *Wheat Belly,* calls today's wheat "frankenwheat," which is not the same wheat that our grandparents ate. Most whole wheat products today are made from a high-yield hybridized "dwarf" wheat grain composed of different wheat varieties. This new wheat is inflammatory and highly addictive. It contains a protein that is as addictive as drugs, causes us to eat more, and can even lead to other health problems. Dr. Davis explains that eliminating wheat from our diets can "prevent fat storage, shrink unsightly bulges, and reverse many different health problems."

Let's take a closer look at what is in this so-called "frankenwheat":

- ꙮ **Gluten** is a protein in wheat and other grains like barley and rye. Modern wheat breads contain ten times the amount of gluten found in them fifty years ago. According to world-renowned gluten expert Dr. Alessio Fasano, who has published more than 200 peer-reviewed studies on gluten, *no human being has the ability to fully digest and break down gluten.* Therefore, consuming it could be damaging the gut lining, leading to leaky gut. He discovered a protein in gluten called zonulin, which creates inflammation in the gut and the body and is linked to an increase in almost every health condition ranging from cancer to heart disease and beyond. The effects of gluten can be far-reaching and could even be harming our brain. Dr. David Perlmutter, author of *Grain Brain,* says that gluten, wheat, and sugar are prime reasons for many neurological diseases from Alzheimer's to ADHD.

* **Amylopectin-A** is a "super starch" found in modern wheat because of hybridization. According to Dr. Davis, it is this super starch that causes our blood sugar to spike higher than a spoonful of sugar and stimulates our appetite.

* **Polypeptides** are short chain amino acids produced when wheat comes into contact with stomach acids. These polypeptides cross the blood-brain barrier and act like opiates on the brain, which gives us a little "high." Anytime something gives us a high, it can be addictive. There have also been studies linking schizophrenia, autism, and other neurological conditions to wheat and gluten, which could be connected to the polypeptides. More research is needed in this area.

* **Phytic acids** contained in wheat may be another problem. Phytic acids are considered antinutrients since they bind to and uptake minerals preventing the body from absorbing them. Soaking, sprouting, or fermenting grains can remove some of the phytic acids. This is why some people who have trouble with grains can better handle those that have been sprouted or fermented (as in traditional sourdough). *Note that nuts, legumes, soy, and other grains also contain phytic acids. Soy has very high levels of phytic acid, which are not removed with soaking and sprouting, but fermenting does work. That is why fermented soy is the only kind I recommend.*

* **Wheat germ agglutinin (WGA)** is a type of lectin found in wheat. Although gluten tends to get all the glory when it comes to the ill effects of eating wheat, WGA might be one of the main reasons why wheat is causing a myriad of health issues in a growing number of people. Lectins are like natural pesticides designed to protect its host from predators and pests. But it turns out that these substances can accumulate in tissues and wreak havoc on those of us who consume them. According to Dr. Joseph Mercola, WGA has been found in studies to send out pro-inflammatory messages, damage the gut lining, interfere with white blood cell function, and it also can cross the blood

brain barrier attacking the myelin sheath. Very resistant to breakdown, sprouting does not seem to remove the WGA either.

❧ The modern dwarf wheat plant is capable of producing up to 23,000 **different proteins,** all of which could potentially create immune responses. There is some evidence that ancient forms of wheat (such as einkorn or kamut), because they are not hybridized, may not negatively impact health to the same degree that our modern wheat does.

We are just beginning to scratch the surface when it comes to understanding the impact that whole wheat, gluten, and even other grains could have on our health. Much more research is needed. But all of this begs the question: should anyone be eating modern whole wheat? Certainly those with digestive issues, blood sugar issues, diabetes, excess weight, chronic inflammation/arthritis, heart disease, neurological issues, or autoimmune disease might do well to ditch the wheat, and possibly all grains.

CELIAC DISEASE

It is estimated that about 1 percent of the population has a very serious autoimmune reaction to gluten called celiac disease. According to celiac expert Dr. Alessio Fasano, you need to carry the genetic predisposition for celiac disease, and then an environmental trigger that "turns on the disease." People who have celiac disease MUST always avoid gluten and ingredients that contain gluten. Even minuscule amounts can lead to debilitating symptoms and permanent damage to the gut lining. People with celiac disease should even avoid products that could have cross-contamination from gluten. Some of the possible complications associated with celiac disease include short stature/failure to thrive, osteoporosis, anemia, fertility issues, malnutrition, increased risk of cancer, neurological issues, autoimmune disorders, type 1 diabetes, thyroid issues, heart disease, and digestive diseases. Because celiac disease can be life-threatening, it is important to rule it out if you suspect gluten is causing you trouble. *Many of the same complications can also arise from a non-celiac gluten sensitivity as well.*

Dairy

Dairy is as wholesome as apple pie. Milk, cheese, and ice cream are dietary staples. They are comforting and delicious. But what if milk isn't really doing your body good? There are three different components of dairy that we could be reacting to:

- **Lactose.** The most common issue with dairy is an inability to digest the lactose, which is a disaccharide sugar molecule which makes up about 2–8 percent of milk. It is estimated that only about 40 percent of the population produces the enzymes needed to properly digest lactose. That means that for the majority of the population, milk products work against our digestion/metabolism. The classic symptoms of lactose intolerance affect the digestive tract (constipation, diarrhea, gas, bloating, pain), the skin (rashes, itching, eczema), and also the urinary tract (bed-wetting, leaking).

  But is it really the milk we have a problem with, or what is done to process it? Milk in its raw state naturally contains the enzymes needed to digest lactose. Pasteurizing, which involves heating the milk, kills these natural components. That is why some people with lactose issues may be able to handle raw milk. In fact, raw organic milk may be very healing to the digestion.

- **Casein.** Another compound that people can react to in dairy is the protein casein. People with a casein allergy can have quite serious reactions including vomiting, hives, or difficulty breathing. The response to a casein intolerance, however, can be delayed including joint pain, fatigue, or mood, behavior, and neurological symptoms. Casein sensitivity has been implicated in autism, ADHD, and even type 1 diabetes. When broken down, casein releases opiate-like compounds called casomorphins, which can cross the blood brain barrier and create an additive reaction similar to wheat peptides.

  It turns out that not all cows produce the same kind of casein. Dairy from Holstein cows, the type from which most of the dairy in the United States is produced, contains the A1 casein. The jury is still out on the difference, but some claim that the

A2 casein, produced by Jersey cows, may not provoke the same reactions as the A1 protein does. Milk from goats and sheep does not contain A1 casein, possibly explaining why it may be tolerated better.

- ❧ **Whey.** A combination of proteins and peptides, this is the liquidy stuff that remains when cheese is made or that collects on the top of your yogurt. Whey protein is a staple for a lot of athletes and bodybuilders (I recommend always getting grass-fed if you do tolerate and choose whey), but is another protein that can create a reaction for some.

Milk and Hormones

Another reason to consider ditching the dairy is the hormones. All milk, even organic and grass-fed varieties, contains hormones. They are naturally present in dairy. But conventional factory-farmed milk also contains the hormones given to cows to increase milk production and prevent infection. One potential risk factor that drinking dairy increases is the promotion of insulin-like growth factor-1 (IGF-1), which has been linked in several different studies to cancer. According to a 2009 study conducted at Dartmouth, "a potent link to dairy seems to exist for three hormone-responsive glands. Acne, breast cancer and prostate cancer have all been linked epidemiologically to dairy intake."

Milk and Our Bones

You might be thinking, "But don't I need milk for strong bones?" Despite all those celebrities with milk mustaches telling us that milk "does a body good," studies show that countries with the highest milk consumption also have the highest rates of fractures and osteoporosis. The Harvard Nurses' Health Study following 78,000 women for a twelve-year period found that milk did not protect against bone fractures. In fact, those who drank three glasses per day had more fractures than those who rarely drank milk.

Here is the thing: Calcium is important for our bones, but it can't work alone. I like to explain it this way: Imagine that you are moving. You hire a moving company that sends only one person to do all the lifting. Sure, he will be able to move the small items, but he can only lift one side of a long couch or mattress. Similarly, in order for calcium to do its job, it needs the key "cofactors"—the helpers—that move it into the bones. These cofactors include magnesium, vitamin D3, vitamin K, and trace minerals. Milk does not supply all of these in the ideal ratios for getting calcium into the bones. But even worse for our bones than drinking milk is taking cheap calcium supplements that are made from poorly absorbed forms of calcium, without the cofactors. Calcium that is not absorbed can end up in the arteries and kidneys, creating calcifications where they are not supposed to be. Some nondairy foods that support strong bones include sardines, canned salmon, bok choy, broccoli, kale, sesame seeds (or tahini), chia seeds, figs, legumes, almonds, seaweed. If you are looking for a good calcium supplement, I recommend a product called AlgaeCal, which has a highly absorbable algae-based form of calcium and also contains the necessary cofactors for absorption.

Dairy is acidifying and mucus-producing in the body, which works against bone building. When the body is too acidic, calcium is needed to "buffer" the acidity, so it will be diverted from the bones to offset excess acid in the bloodstream.

Below are some reasons to consider going dairy-free:

- Digestive troubles—both constipation and loose stools
- "Seasonal" allergies, which can often be improved through nutritional changes like giving up dairy
- Chronic sinus infections, frequent ear infections in kids, and frequent croup or asthma
- Bed-wetting and leaking, which I have seen corrected almost overnight by giving up the dairy
- Focus and attention problems, which may be linked to milk sensitivity in some kids
- Frequent fractures or poor healing
- Heart disease, hormonal issues, and kidney stones, which all may be at least partially linked to dairy intolerance

Wait! What about Butter?

Butter, when sourced from organic grass-fed cows, is a "good fat." But it is also dairy-based. If you like, ghee is a good alternative because it is clarified butter, which removes all but a tiny trace of the milk proteins. Only those who are highly dairy sensitive will have an issue with ghee. Even butter may be tolerated by certain people with milder dairy intolerance issues because of the higher fat content; only about 1 percent of butter is comprised of protein (milk solids), which is what causes the reaction.

Genetically Modified Foods

Another group of foods that could be contributing to poor gut health and food intolerances is GMOs (genetically modified organisms). GMOs are created by forcing DNA material/proteins from another organism (such as insects, other plants, animals, viruses) into the DNA of a plant. This process essentially creates a new genome for that modified plant, which would not be able to occur in nature.

This is a highly contentious topic. Proponents say that genetic modification benefits include enhancing crop productivity, enabling farmers to create crops that are naturally resistant to insects, producing larger plants more quickly, and the like. Using that logic, I can understand how the lobbyists were able to sell the federal government on GMOs initially. But questions are arising about the impact on our health, the environment, and whether they even work.

Perhaps one of the least likely and earliest activists to speak out against GMOs was Pope John Paul II, who believed that GMOs went against God's will. In the year 2000, he spoke to 50,000 farmers urging them to "resist the temptation of high productivity and profit that work to the detriment of nature. When farmers forget this basic principle and become tyrants of the earth rather than its custodians, sooner or later the earth rebels."

Are They Safe?

The Food and Drug Administration (FDA) has found "no evidence" that GMOs present any health problems and has ruled them as GRAS (generally recognized as safe). However, the FDA did admit that there could be some unforeseeable issues with them: "Virtually all known allergens are proteins. Since genetic engineering can introduce a new protein into a food plant, it is possible that this technique could introduce a previously unknown allergen into the food supply or into a new food. A second possible problem is the introduction of toxins into the food crop. A third possible issue is the introduction of anti-nutrients."

Despite the fact that there have been numerous peer-reviewed studies showing that GMOs are essentially safe, a 2012 French study came to some very different conclusions. The study followed 200 rats, some of which were fed GMO corn, and others non-GMO corn. The study lasted two years (the life span of a rat), which is much longer than the typical ninety-day length of other studies. The researchers found that rats fed a diet of GMO corn were more likely than controls to develop tumors, organ damage, and die prematurely. Generally, these consequences happened after ninety days, which would have been out of the scope of previous studies. This study faced numerous criticisms and was eventually retracted. Some of the criticisms included that the population was not large enough and was prone to develop tumors, the results were not dose-dependent, and the researchers were not unbiased. More research is needed to look at the impact of GMOs, but if there were no foreseeable downsides, why have twenty-six countries banned them?

How Do You Know iaf a Food Is Genetically Modified?

Until labeling is required by law, U.S. manufacturers do not have to tell us if their product contains GMO ingredients or not. Some companies believe we have the right to know what is in our food and are adding the Non-GMO Project label to show GMOs are not utilized anywhere in their production chain. The certified organic label also tells you that the product does not contain GMO ingredients.

Crops Likely to Be GMO (estimated percent to be GMO):

1. *Soy (94 percent)*

2. *Corn (88 percent)*

3. *Canola (90 percent)*

4. *Sugar from sugar beets (95 percent)*

5. *Cotton, cottonseed oil (90 percent)*

6. *Zucchini, summer squash (25,000 acres)*

SOURCE: NON-GMO PROJECT, 2011

Buying organic or certified non-GMO for the above foods is the only way to be sure you are not getting GMOs. The other way GMOs are making their way into our diets is via animals fed GMOs crops (alfalfa, soy, corn). This changes the nutritional profile and potentially the allergenic potential of foods from those animals. Choosing organic and grass-fed sources for our animal proteins means we avoid GMOs, antibiotics, hormones, etc.

Soy is a special case. In addition to being one of the top GMO foods, soy has some other considerable downsides. Companies add soy as a cheap protein source to many foods to increase the protein content. Many restaurants also use it since it is an inexpensive and neutral-tasting oil. It is utilized frequently in vegan diets as meat and dairy replacements. But because soy has the highest content of phytic acids—which bind to and uptake minerals—of any food, it can lead to mineral depletion. Poorly digested, soy might contribute to a leaky gut and other digestive issues. Genistein, a protein in soy, is a natural phytoestrogen, meaning it mimics estrogen in humans. There is quite a debate going on about whether or not that is a good thing. In some studies, genistein appears to compete with bad estrogens, which is considered positive. Yet, because it introduces estrogens into the body, that can be viewed as negative, especially for babies and children. According to Dr. Mercola, "infants fed soy formula take in an estimated three to five birth control pills' worth of estrogen every day." And according to a study published in *Environmental Health Perspectives*, babies fed soy formula had an increased risk of uterine fibroids later in life. Soy is also a goitrogen and linked to thyroid issues, so anyone with thyroid issues would do well to avoid it entirely. As you can see, there is considerable evidence pointing to the fact that soy is not a health food. Because it is in so many processed foods, the more processed the diet is, the harder it is to avoid.

GMOs' Environmental Impact

The evidence is mounting that GMOs may be having a negative impact on our environment—including killing off bees and butterflies, which could be disastrous for the high percentage of important crops relying on bees for pollination. It appears that GMO seeds can infect non-GMO crops, so it is possible that we might not be able to avoid them in the very near future, short of giving up that food entirely.

Do They Even Work?

The ultimate kicker is that insects are evolving and some GMOs are starting to fail to provide the promised protection from pests! So increasing amounts of pesticides need to be used on many GMO crops.

Those in the business of GMOs obviously want us to believe there are no health issues. GMOs are big business. The science is still very young on this issue. There simply needs to be more research. My take is that until there are definitive answers about the long-term implications of GMOs for humans, consuming them might just make us unwitting participants in a giant science experiment. *There are many books and documentaries dedicated to genetic modification. If you are interested in learning more about GMOs, check the resources section at the back of this book.*

Eggs—Should I Give Them Up?

Eggs are an excellent source of protein and choline, which is good for our brain. Eggs also contain lutein and zeaxanthin, which are important for our eye health. A breakfast of eggs offers stable blood sugar and lasting energy, a good choice for a healthy metabolism. But some people react very poorly to eggs, so they are optional to remove. You might want to give them a break if you suspect that you have an issue with eggs, suffer from gallbladder trouble, or simply want to be as thorough as possible on the elimination. Others might decide to keep eggs in and see how they feel.

If you do choose to keep eggs in your diet, make sure you get organic or non-GMO certified eggs. It would be even better if you can find pastured eggs. Pastured chickens are allowed to forage and eat their natural diet, which includes bugs and grass. Chickens with higher-quality healthier diets produce more nutritious eggs that are higher in omega-3s and therefore less inflammatory. Do a side-by-side comparison of a pastured egg and a conventional egg, and notice how dark orange in color the pastured yolk is compared to the conventional egg—that is an indication of the higher nutrient content. Yes, they are more expensive, but you get what you pay for, right? Pay the grocer now or the doctor later.

If you choose to eliminate eggs, you can still enjoy certain recipes that require them. Just make an egg replacer out of chia seeds! Mix one tablespoon of chia seeds (or ground flax) with three tablespoons water, and let hydrate. That will fill in for an egg in a recipe!

HORMONE HIGHLIGHT: THYROID HORMONES

No discussion of metabolism would be complete without mentioning the thyroid, the starter for our metabolic engine.

A butterfly-shaped organ sitting just below the Adam's apple, the thyroid produces the hormones responsible for a wide range of functions, including the heart and nervous system operation, regulating body temperature, energy production and use, muscle function and strength, menstrual cycle/hormones, and even cognitive functioning.

One of the keys to thyroid health is good gut health. An underlying infection, low digestive fire, or a leaky gut can wreak havoc on our thyroid. Other things that can impact the thyroid are pesticides, heavy metals, chlorine, stress, and nutritional deficiencies. Food intolerances can be a problem (especially gluten, soy, and goitrogens). According to gluten expert Dr. Tom O'Bryan in *The Thyroid Sessions*, "43% of people with a sensitivity to gluten will manifest some type of thyroid dysfunction." It is no wonder that an estimated 50 million people suffer from a thyroid issue, many of which are undiagnosed. Thyroid cancer is also now one of the fastest growing cancers.

More likely to affect women, classic low thyroid symptoms include low body temperature, dry skin or hair, sluggish digestion/constipation, foggy brain, fatigue, depression, weight gain, fluid retention, enlarged thyroid gland, low sex drive, and thinning eyebrows (on the outer corner).

There is a yin and yang to the thyroid. If the thyroid is underactive, the metabolism will slow down, which can also lead to hormone issues and weight gain. If the thyroid is overactive, meaning it is making (or someone is taking) too many thyroid hormones, it can cause weight loss, bulging eyes, anxiety, sweating, heat intolerance, irregular heartbeat, light sensitivity, bone loss, and an enlarged thyroid gland. Autoimmune disorders can lead to a combination overactive/underactive thyroid.

Are You Eating Too Much Kale or Broccoli?

Goitrogens are some of the healthiest foods on earth, with powerful cancer-fighting compounds. But in some people, they could be interfering with and enlarging your thyroid gland. Goitrogens include cabbage, spinach, kale, brussels sprouts, cauliflower, canola, radishes, turnips, collards, broccoli, bok choy, rutabagas, peanuts, peaches, pine nuts, strawberries, watercress, and—perhaps worst of all—gluten and soy.

It is not clear if everyone with thyroid issues needs to avoid goitrogens. However, for those concerned about their thyroid, gently cooking or steaming goitrogens first might reduce the effect.

Other ways to support the thyroid gland nutritionally:

- Assess and treat the gut for infection or leaky gut.

- Identify food intolerances (particularly gluten and soy).

- Get plenty of rest and fluids.

- Limit (or eliminate) raw goitrogenic foods (many green smoothies and juices contain raw goitrogens).

- Make sure to obtain the *right amount* of iodine in the diet. The best food sources of iodine are sea vegetables, especially kelp. *Note: increasing iodine consumption can worsen thyroid problems for some individuals, especially those with autoimmune thyroid issues. Find a qualified health practitioner to discuss your specific case.*

- Selenium is important for thyroid health and cancer prevention. You can get your daily amount with most multivitamins, or about four to five Brazil nuts a day—one of the best sources. *But don't eat too many Brazil nuts because the body only needs trace amounts of selenium, and you can actually get too much!*

- Avoid pesticides, heavy metals, and chlorine.

- Some might find that supporting the thyroid with an adaptogenic herb is useful (adaptogens do exactly what their name suggests, they help the body adapt to and deal with stress).

Ashwagandha is an excellent choice. *Consult your physician to see if this is right for you.*

If you suspect you might have thyroid issues or have not had your thyroid checked recently, it might be time to schedule a visit with a qualified health care practitioner trained in the area of thyroid health who can help you diagnose and treat thyroid disorders.

Is Grain-Free or Paleo Right for Me?

One of the hottest new nutrition trends is based on the oldest way of eating ever—the way of the Paleolithic people or the hunter-gatherers, referred to as "Paleo." In the Paleolithic era, there was no agriculture, so there were no grains. There were obviously no refined sugars or flours and no pasteurization. People who follow the Paleo approach avoid grains, sugars, pasteurized dairy, and legumes—just as the cavemen did.

Since these foods are big culprits in our unexplained weight gain and health issues, many people might find that the Paleo approach brings positive results for weight loss, improved energy, focus, and much more. Those who are suffering from autoimmune conditions often find that their health improves.

If you want to give Paleo a try, in addition to the other foods you will want to remove all grains and legumes during the elimination phase. You can reintroduce them in phase three, one by one to see if you have a reaction. Because each of us is an individual, I recommend exploring your options and determining which approach works best for you. Some people might find that sprouting or fermenting grains and legumes works best for them.

If you want to learn more about Paleo, check the references section at the back of the book. There is a plethora of good books and online resources to give you more information. Even if you do not go 100 percent Paleo, incorporating some grain-free recipes into your regular diet is an excellent option.

So How Do You Know If You Are Reacting to a Food?

On an elimination diet, you remove foods and then bring them back one at a time. This enables people to become more tuned in to reactions. Some reactions will be immediate or extreme (like digestive pain, bloating, runny nose, tickle in the throat, coughing or sneezing fits, or itchiness), and others may be delayed or vague (fatigue, sluggishness, moodiness, brain fog, muscle aches/pains, sleep issues, anxiety, weight gain). You might also find that you are not reacting to, and are okay with, certain foods.

Why Am I Reacting?

When someone reacts to a food, the next question I often get is: "Why am I reacting to this food that I have eaten my whole life without any trouble?" Food intolerances can develop very gradually over years. The reactions can be very vague and sneaky. Our bodies works hard to cope with the symptoms, so just because you never noticed a reaction to a food before does not mean you might not have been reacting to it. Or maybe you had been taking Advil in bulk for years like I did.

Food intolerances are rooted in the gut. One of the main reasons we are seeing a rise in food intolerances is because there is a rise in leaky gut.

Leaky Gut: When What Happens in Vegas Doesn't Stay There

Remember that one of the jobs of our intestinal wall is to be a bouncer—to keep the riffraff (bacteria, toxins, proteins) out and let the good guys (nutrients) in. When our intestinal wall is healthy, it has tight junctures that ensure that particles that are supposed to stay within our intestines stay there. But when we have a leaky gut, things that are not supposed to be outside the intestines (like partially digested proteins, toxins) can leak out into the bloodstream and create inflammation and other symptoms. This leaking can cause our immune system to go haywire.

Many different things can cause a leaky gut: viral or bacterial infection, parasite, GMOs, food intolerances, as well as antibiotic, steroid, or frequent NSAID (like Advil) use. So it turns out that I wasn't just numbing my pain, I might have been making my leaky gut worse by popping Advil all those years!

When someone discovers that they are reacting to a food, the next questions I usually get are the following.

Do I Have to Avoid It Forever?

The good news is that food intolerances are not always permanent. The answer to whether or not a food needs to be avoided forever comes down to the classic chicken or the egg question: Which came first the gut issue or the food intolerance?

If the food intolerance caused the gut health issue, then the answer is more likely to be: avoid it for life. But if the gut health imbalance caused the food intolerance, the answer is more likely to be: remove the food for a period of time, heal the gut, and then perhaps the food can be tolerated again. We may not always be sure which one came first, but we need to treat them both at the same time (remove the offending food and support the gut to heal). Later, we will look at how to eliminate foods and heal the gut.

The one possible exception to this rule is gluten. Because the symptoms of gluten sensitivity can be so subtle, almost silent, many people will have no idea they are reacting to it at all. Also, because no one really is able to digest it and it can contribute to gut inflammation, my personal take on gluten is that *everyone, even those not reacting in an obvious way,* can benefit from *at the very least* cutting back on gluten and wheat.

Should I Be Tested for Food Intolerance?

A food elimination diet/food challenge is a good place to start, but it may not just be gluten, soy, or dairy causing your chronic migraines, aching joints, fatigue, skin rashes, and digestion issues. If you do not get relief from a food elimination diet—or if you just want to cut to the chase and get the data—you might want to invest in a food intolerance test. I have seen almost anything show up on a food intolerance panel including foods that are not normally removed in a food elimination diet—such as potatoes, rice, bananas, artichoke, beef, squash, coffee, strawberries, oranges, and even vanilla and cinnamon. I use Alcat Laboratories to identify food intolerances.

The Bottom Line: Ignorance Isn't Bliss

There is a mental, emotional, and physical component to giving up foods and changing habits. Some of the things I am suggesting that you eliminate are the very foods and drinks you *love* to eat every single day. We might even be physically and mentally addicted to them. It is not uncommon to doubt that you can even function without these foods. This is one of the key reasons that people don't want to try an elimination diet—because they don't want to give key foods up, so they think they'd rather not know.

But ignorance is not always bliss.

Is that slice of toast in the morning really worth it if it's leading to your weight gain and other serious health issues? If you have a long and growing list of chronic health complaints, you could have a food intolerance.

In part two of this book, you will be guided through an elimination diet to help you identify food intolerances with recipes provided to help you put it into practice. This can be a really big shift! Take your time and do your best. Just remember that knowledge is power. If there is a food standing between you and vibrant health, wouldn't you want to know about it?

⚜ 5 ⚜

Lose the Toxic Weight
Toxins Tell Our Bodies to Store Fat and Promote Disease

We should stop counting calories and start counting chemicals.

—UNKNOWN

Having a healthy metabolism means that our digestion is working, our hormones are communicating, and our bodies are able to nourish our cells and remove the waste effectively. Toxins get in the way and interrupt our hormones and a healthy metabolism.

In its infinite wisdom, the human body has multiple systems in place that are designed to keep us healthy and protect us from harm. Similar to the mechanisms for dealing with blood sugar, we come equipped with multiple detoxification organs and systems designed to safely remove and clear toxic substances from the body. When the body can't remove them all, it stores them in the safest place away from our brain and organs. Yep, you guessed it, in our fat. This creates toxic fat, which is harder to lose because the body wants to keep harmful substances safely insulated from our organs. The more toxins we introduce into our diet and environment, the more likely our body's detox channels won't be able to handle them, and they will accumulate in our adipose tissue.

Case Study: MSG

There are certain toxins that communicate with our bodies and tell them to store more fat—referred to as "obesogens." Hailed as a flavor enhancer, monosodium glutamate (MSG) was introduced to the United States in 1947 and has since been added to many processed, packaged, and fast foods. Although it might make food taste better, it doesn't make us feel so great. In 1969, the journal *Science* published an article that reported on the symptoms of MSG, ranging from headaches to swelling, burning, and more. These symptoms were collectively called "Chinese Food Syndrome," because at the time, most Chinese restaurants were using MSG so liberally in their food it could leave people with headaches.

More recent studies have revealed another symptom of MSG to be weight gain, which is why it is considered an "obesogen." When scientists need overweight rats for a study, they know that MSG will make them gain weight. When rats are injected with MSG, it increases their hunger and creates insulin resistance—a double whammy that leads to prediabetes and rapid weight gain.

Foods "enhanced" with MSG are also highly addictive. Once we start eating them, we crave even more, creating a vicious cycle. The scary thing is that many foods marketed directly at kids are loaded with MSG! It's no wonder we have a childhood obesity problem, considering we start our kids on obesogens at an early age.

Food manufacturers know we are reading labels, so they might try to hide MSG under other names like hydrolyzed vegetable protein, sodium hydrogen glutamate, sodium caseinate, and dozens of other options. Another place where MSG is lurking is in many fast-food restaurants.

Other chemicals that are considered obesogens:

BPA—found in many canned goods and plastics (especially those with the number 3 or 7)

High fructose corn syrup

Phthalates—chemicals found in fragrance products and vinyl products

Perfluorooctanoic acid (PFOA)—found in Teflon pans, microwave popcorn bags, and even pizza boxes

Aspartame—found in "diet" drinks and foods

Getting Rid of Toxic Fat

In order to safely and effectively rid the body of toxic fat, we need to take two basic steps.

1. Stop Introducing New Toxins

We might not see them or think about them much, but we are exposed to toxins via air, land, water, and our food. Below are some possible ways that toxins can sneak into our world:

- Chemicals in your shampoo, in the laundry detergent that you washed your sheets in, in your makeup, and on your dry-cleaned clothes

- Toxins that you breathe in at your office, inside your new car, and outside during your run or from air fresheners and candles

- Chemicals on your nonstick cookware and in the artificial sweetener you added to your coffee

- Pesticides on your morning fruit and lunchtime salad

- Mercury in your canned tuna fish

- Heavy metals in our water supply and food

- Chemicals like MSG, preservatives, and artificial colors that are added to our foods

- Artificial flavors and colors in sports drinks, sodas, candies, and even pickles

- Cellular radiation from your cellphone and other WiFi technology

- Radiation emitted from nuclear disasters like the one in Fukushima, automobiles, the sun, x-rays, mammograms, and confined animal feedlots

- Bisphenol-A (BPAs) in the plastic water bottles, plastic wrap, cans, and grocery store receipts we are handed

- Toxins on the inside of your fast-food containers and microwave popcorn bags

It might sound too simple, but one of the best things we can do to detoxify the body is to just eat more whole, real foods. According to a study published in *Environmental Health Perspectives*, by avoiding canned foods and plastic containers and consuming a whole foods diet for just three days, participating families were able to reduce the BPAs in their urine by 60 percent, and some lowered them by 75 percent. That was just in three days!

Have you heard the advice "shop the perimeter of the store"? The perimeter is where you will find more whole, fresh foods and fewer packaged and processed ones. Eating fewer packaged and processed foods and more fresh whole foods is probably the simplest way to reduce our exposure to chemicals and toxins. Choosing organic for the foods that are more likely to be contaminated with pesticides, hormones, and antibiotics and avoiding GMOs is also very useful.

Is Organic Really Worth It?

Have you ever found yourself standing in the produce section of the grocery store wondering if the organic strawberries are really worth paying more for than the conventional ones? There are a number of reasons why organic is more expensive, ranging from the added cost for the certifications to the extra work it takes to protect crops from insects without the use of pesticides and rotating the crops to ensure higher-quality soils. In the case of animal proteins, it costs more to raise animals to graze on pastures, and also not use any antibiotics, hormones, or GMO feed. But is all this extra effort worth it? Let's take a look at plant-based foods first.

Produce

The soil is our external metabolism. It must be free of pesticides and herbicides for the body to heal.

—MAX GERSON, MD

According to a 2005 report by the College of Agriculture and Life Sciences at Cornell, there is "ample evidence that pesticides present a threat to human health." The health impact of pesticides includes cancer as well as neurological, respiratory, and reproductive issues. Worldwide, about three billion pesticides are used each year. The majority of foods in U.S. supermarkets have detectable levels of pesticide residues. For certain crops (strawberries, apples, celery, peaches, pears), 90 percent were found to contain pesticides. Apples had thirty-seven different pesticides!

The good news is that according to a study published in the journal *Environmental Research*, eating organic for just one week can reduce exposure to pesticides by close to 90 percent.

So ideally, buying organic for all produce is the safest way to go. But for those who are trying to save a little bit of money, let's take a closer look at when it is really important to spring for the organic version, and when it might be okay to stick with the conventional ones. One general question to use is do you eat or peel off the skin? Foods like bananas and avocados that have a fairly thick skin protecting the fruit are less likely to be contaminated. But for delicate fruit like strawberries and leafy greens, it is worth it to spring for organic. The Environmental Working Group (EWG) came up with a list of produce most likely to be contaminated, called the Dirty Dozen, to help us know when to pay extra for organic:

The 2014 EWG Dirty Dozen (Plus)

1. Apples
2. Strawberries
3. Grapes
4. Celery
5. Peaches
6. Spinach
7. Sweet bell peppers
8. Nectarines (imported)
9. Cucumbers
10. Cherry tomatoes
11. Snap peas (imported)
12. Potatoes

Plus:

13. Hot peppers
14. Blueberries (domestic)
15. Lettuce
16. Kale/ collard greens

—THE ENVIRONMENTAL WORKING GROUP (EWG). 2014.
The Dirty Dozen Plus is updated annually. Visit *www.ewg.org* to see the full rankings of produce. You can also download a PDF version or an app that lists the Dirty Dozen so you can carry the latest and greatest info on your phone when you go shopping.

If you shop at farmers markets, get to know the growers, and ask them about their practices. Some will explain that the produce is grown organically, but they do not have the organic seal. Go for it anyway. It is expensive to get and maintain organic certification, so small growers will often choose not to certify, even though they use organic growing practices.

Note: I always recommend using 100 percent organic produce if you are juicing it or making tea (such as the detoxing artichoke tea in the recipe section). In each glass of juice, there are typically several pounds of produce!

Animal Proteins

When you eat animal proteins (such as eggs, chicken, pork, beef, dairy), always keep in mind that you are consuming the diet the animal ate. Conventionally raised animals eat inexpensive feed made from corn, soy, and other grains—a diet designed to fatten them up. This feed may have been treated with pesticides or could be genetically modified. They also regularly receive antibiotics to increase their growth and inhibit the spread of bacteria due to tight living conditions. Over 80 percent of all antibiotics in the United States are fed to conventional wild stock; this amounts to close to thirty million pounds. According to the EWG, this has led to documented levels of resistant bacterial strains in 81 percent of ground turkey, 69 percent of pork chops, 55 percent of ground beef, and 39 percent of chicken meat. The World Health Organization says that excessive use of antibiotics in livestock is contributing to a resistance that could create a dangerous "post-antibiotic era" when infections caused by bacteria, parasites, viruses, and fungi can no longer be treated with existing medications.

Many conventional animals are also given growth hormones like rBGH and rBST, which are designed to make them grow bigger faster. One other chemical that animals are given to promote growth is ractopamine. Used in 80 percent of conventional U.S. cattle and pig operations, ractopamine is banned in Europe, China, Russia, and many other countries. The European Food Safety Authority indicates that ractopamine causes "elevated heart rates and heart-pounding sensations in humans"; these symptoms are also documented in animal studies.

Free-range and organic animals are allowed to roam and graze on grass, the diet that they are designed to eat. Because their diet is healthier, their meat and other products are healthier. Grass-fed organic proteins are naturally higher in omega-3s, which reduce inflammation, whereas conventional meats and eggs are higher in omega-6s, which promote inflammation (see chapter six on inflammation to learn more). So when it comes to animal proteins, it is worth every penny to buy organic and free-range/pasture-raised for *all* animal-based products. Some restaurants and other establishments are starting to recognize the demand for non-GMO and organic meats and other products.

Heavy Metals: Lead, Cadmium, Mercury, and Aluminum

Heavy metals are found in our air, soil, water, and food in larger amounts than ever before and can present a serious threat to human health. According to Dr. Steven Schechter, toxins like radiation and heavy metals can be "trapped in the body and produce cumulative long-term effects."

The farther up an animal is on the food chain, the more likely toxins can build up. So in the case of fish, a large fish like shark and tuna that has lived longer and had more exposures to toxins in its environment and diet is more likely to carry more mercury and other toxins than a smaller fish that is not as old, like a sardine or herring. So if you enjoy fish, it is important to choose the lower mercury fish.

Some organic metals act as nutrients in the body in the right amounts, including copper, zinc, and manganese. But if too much of these metals are taken in, they can lead to health problems. Then there are the non-organic heavy metals that are found in our air, soil, water, and food that have accumulated from pesticide use.

One way we can fight against heavy metal accumulation is to do our best to avoid the sources, but this might not always be possible, because it is not always obvious where they are hiding. Another tactic is to ensure that our bodies are not minerally deficient. When the body has the optimal amount of minerals and metals, those offer a protection against the uptake of toxins. This is called "selective uptake," according to Dr. Steven Schechter in *Fighting Radiation and Chemical Pollutants*. For example, optimal serum levels of iodine can block the body from taking up certain radioactive isotopes, according to Schechter.

Plastics and Cans

Consuming a lot of foods and drinks from plastic bottles or metal cans exposes the body to BPAs, which can be harmful to the hormones and metabolism and have even been linked to certain cancers. Substances leaching out of plastic food packaging materials can act as functional estrogens and contribute to obesity, according to research published in *Environmental Health Perspective*.

Some tips:

- Do not microwave anything in plastic containers or bags (in fact, do not microwave when you have an alternative).

- Drink water and other beverages from a glass container or stainless steel whenever possible.

- Opt for fresh, dried, or boxed foods when possible, in place of canned goods.

- BPAs are on cash register receipts too, so if you have the option, get your receipt electronically.

Radiation

We are continually exposed to radiation from both natural and artificial sources. One example of natural radiation would be the sun's rays. In small amounts, sunlight actually offers a health benefit. Approximately twenty minutes of sun daily boosts the body's production of vitamin D, which is a powerful immune system regulator. But too much radiation from the sun can lead to the formation of free radicals. So it is good to get a small amount of unprotected sun most days of the week but to use protective clothing and/or a mineral-based sunscreen if you plan to be out longer.

We are also exposed to radiation from cellphones and other technology. There have been some reports of a fairly new breast cancer that is emerging in young girls located underneath the armpit, along the bra line. Although the link is not yet proven, it is hypothesized that this could be from carrying their cellphones in the side of their bras. Until more is known about cellular radiation, we should try to keep our cellular devices away from our bodies whenever possible—using a headset when we talk, carrying them in a purse or other bag when not in use.

Skin Care Products and Detergents

What we put on our skin and hair ends up inside our body as well. So it is important to use nontoxic soaps, shampoos, laundry detergents, and skin care and makeup products. Below is a partial list of ingredients that are best to avoid; visit the EWG website for a full list:

- BHA (butylated hydroxyanisole)
- Sulfates (sodium lauryl sulfate [SLS] or ammonium lauryl sulfate)
- Parabens
- Chemical propylene glycol

- Triclosan
    - Ethoxylates and dioxane
    - Nitrosamine
    - Methyl, propyl, butyl, and ethyl paraben
    - Triethanolamine (TEA)/diethanolamine (DEA)
    - Artificial dyes and colors
    - Zirconium, benzalkonium chloride, bismuth, antimony, barium sulfate, aluminum, tin, chromium, benzene, and PCBs
    - Synthetic fragrances/phthalates. Avoid personal care products listing "perfume" or "fragrance" in the ingredients, which is a broad term that often signals phthalate ingredients. Phthalates are found in scented candles, laundry detergent, and many other personal care products. Phthalates are plasticizing, hormone-disrupting chemicals dubbed "obesogens" for their likely ability to promote weight gain. A study also found that people with higher levels of phthalates in their bodies were twice as likely to have diabetes.
    - Look for sunscreens without oxybenzone, a synthetic chemical that absorbs the sun's rays but also readily penetrates the skin. It can disrupt natural hormones and cause allergic reactions.
    - Although it appears to be a safe ingredient for antiaging night creams, it is best to avoid sunscreens or makeup that list "retinyl palmitate" or "retinol palmitate" (a form of vitamin A), which has been shown to increase tumor growth when used on skin that is exposed to sunlight. The safest option is to choose mineral-based makeups and sunscreens, because they do not have chemicals.)

2. Support the Body's Detoxification Channels

Not bringing in new toxins is a good start, and studies show that consciously avoiding certain toxins like BPAs (by not eating from cans and plastics) can result in a measurable reduction of the toxin in the body within days. The next step is to support the body in ushering out existing toxins that have accumulated.

Let's take a look at the different detoxification organs and systems and how we can help them to remove toxins and chemicals and repair cellular damage.

Digestive System/The Colon

As we learned in chapter three, the digestive system is central to our health and metabolism. In order to properly detoxify, it is critical for the digestive system to be working and removing waste—and that means a daily bowel movement (BM). If the digestive system is not eliminating well, we could be reabsorbing toxins to be released back into the bloodstream. So making sure that food waste is being effectively eliminated is critical for all people wanting to lose weight or detoxify the body. Review chapter three for some tips for optimizing digestion and elimination.

The Skin

The largest organ in the human body, our skin plays a very important role in detoxification and can be a "window" on our internal health. Acne, eczema, rashes, psoriasis, broken capillaries, redness or rosacea, and other conditions of the skin can all be the body trying to tell us that something underneath is amiss. Rather than putting on acne cream or taking a pill, we might want to consider cleaning up our diet first or looking for a food intolerance.

We can support detoxification through the skin in several ways:

- Skin brushing is an ancient art and stimulates the body to detoxify.

- Epsom/sea salt baths help to pull toxins out via the skin.

- Sweating is another way that the body releases toxins via the skin: exercising to a sweat or sitting in a sauna encourages detoxification though the skin. Infrared saunas are the best kind with powerful healing and detoxifying properties.

The Respiratory System

The respiratory system brings in and filters our air, sending oxygen to the bloodstream, where it is carried throughout the body. When we exhale, we are releasing carbon dioxide and other toxins. To support the body, it is important to avoid toxins in the air we breathe: stay away from cigarette smoke (even secondhand), avoid using any chemical-based cleaning products (which can release toxic fumes), and try not to spend time in areas where there are more toxins and particulate matter in the air (like near factories). One way to assist the body to detoxify the respiratory system is by practicing deep breathing, called pranayama in yoga. Even just a couple minutes of quiet deep breathing each day can be useful.

The Kidneys

Every minute, about one quart of blood goes into the kidneys, which filter and eliminate the by-products of metabolism and waste materials from that blood. The kidneys produce red blood cells and play a role in conversion of vitamin D to its active form, which also balances out the calcium levels in the body. They also support the body's balance of fluids and blood pressure by regulating the amount of sodium in the bloodstream and play a big part in regulating our pH balance. Some signs that the kidneys might be under strain? Swelling or edema, urinary tract infections (can be yeast overgrowth as well), and kidney stone formation.

The majority of kidney stones are calcium oxalate stones. *People who are prone to calcium oxalate stones might want to consider a low oxalate diet.* Another type of kidney stone is uric acid, which can result from dehydration, excess protein, or gout.

The following helps the kidneys:

- Avoid dehydration (see chapter nine for more information).
- Avoid sweetened drinks and foods.
- Consume a reasonable amount of protein. Too much protein can put undue strain on the kidneys.
- Avoid NSAIDs if possible.
- Avoid or cut down on caffeine.
- Quit smoking.

The Liver: The Body's Largest Solid Organ Critical for Metabolism, Hormones, and More!

In Chinese medicine, the liver is referred to as the "General of the Army." The largest solid organ in the body, the liver performs over 600 functions including:

- Production of bile for the digestion of fats

- Elimination of excess hormones
- Regulation of blood sugar
- Filtration of the blood
- Absorption, conversion, and storage of fat-soluble vitamins
- Detoxification of substances such as sugars, chemicals, drugs, and even excess hormones.

Everything we take into our body—whether we swallow it, inhale it, or absorb it through our skin—is eventually filtered in the liver. So if the liver is not functioning optimally, it impacts all the other organs and systems in the body, which adds up to hormone imbalances, a sluggish metabolism, and fat accumulation in the liver and the midsection. But the good news is the reverse is also true: strengthening the liver can help to improve the functioning of many other organs, help to balance hormones, and support a healthy metabolism.

It's no wonder in our chemical- and toxin-filled world today that our liver might get overburdened. Fortunately, the liver is amazingly resilient; it is the only organ that, if you cut a chunk off, it literally could regenerate itself from the remaining healthy liver cells. But even the liver has its limits, and if we push it too far, the damage can become permanent. Our liver is critical to our survival. Humans can only live for about two days if the liver fails. So all things considered, it is quite important to occasionally give this organ a much-needed break.

Fatty Liver Disease

Some fat in the liver is normal. But if it exceeds 5 to 10 percent of the liver's total weight, then it is considered a fatty liver (steatosis). Heavy drinking can lead to fatty liver disease. The good news is that fatty liver disease can be reversed in four to six weeks of complete abstinence. If allowed to progress to cirrhosis however, the damage can become permanent. So awareness and early detection are very important.

But alcohol is not the only insult to the liver. In fact, the largest surge in liver disease is actually from nonalcoholic fatty liver disease (NAFLD). It is estimated that 30 percent of Americans have NAFLD (80 percent of obese people). Because there are virtually no symptoms early on, most are completely unaware. Diets high in sugars (especially fructose) and carbs can increase our risk of developing NAFLD, which is probably why 10 percent of children are estimated to have NAFLD (40 percent of obese children).

Although those with NAFLD may have no symptoms, some possible indicators include pain in the upper right abdomen (below the rib cage), weight gain in the midsection, unexplained weight loss, loss of appetite, fatigue, spiderlike blood vessels, itching, fluid retention, allergies, stiff neck, alcohol abuse (or other addictions), malnutrition, nutrient malabsorption, diarrhea, upset stomach, "liver spots," puffy face, hemorrhoids, strong body odor, and chronic throat problems.

The Liver—First Line of Support for Hormones

The liver and our hormones are closely intertwined. The liver manufactures cholesterol—from which all steroid and sex hormones are made. The liver also produces a protein called sex hormone binding globulin (SHBG) responsible for regulating the sex hormones and removing the excess ones. If high levels of estrogen or testosterone are detected, the SHBG protein will bind to it as well as slow down the body's production of that hormone to balance everything out. If the liver is not working optimally and not producing SHBG effectively, it can lead to hormonal imbalances. As one example, excess estrogen might not get removed from the body, which can contribute to estrogen-dominant health problems including endometriosis, fibroids, heavy periods, cysts, infertility, and other symptoms. Excess estrogen also can increase retention of fat around the midsection, and this excess fat is an organ in and of itself producing more fat, which can produce more estrogens, and so on. This is not a good cycle to get into with regard to weight. This condition does not just apply to women; men may experience elevated estrogen levels and declining testosterone levels too. Supporting our liver should be one of the key steps in hormone balancing.

The Liver and B Vitamins

B vitamins are primarily water soluble, so unlike fat-soluble vitamins, the body does not store them for later use. Increased levels of stress, nutrient deficiencies, and absorption issues can all deplete us of the B vitamins. The B vitamins are critical for our metabolism, and the detoxification channels of the liver. Low levels of B vitamins could lead to sluggish detoxification.

The Liver and the Intestines

If your bowel and intestines are not working properly, trying to fix the liver could be troublesome. You might end up running to the bathroom all day long, or if the bowels are not moving, the toxins being released could be reabsorbed. So it is important to clean up the whole digestive system in order to properly support liver function.

The Liver and Emotions

According to traditional Chinese medicine, our emotions can be an indication of the health of our liver. Anger, resentment, frustration, being hard to please, or having a short fuse can all be an indication that the liver needs a little TLC.

Detoxing the Liver

The good news is that the liver has an incredible ability to regenerate and renew if properly supported. To give the liver a much-needed break, try to avoid the following for two to four weeks: alcohol, recreational drugs, sugary foods and drinks, trans fats, refined and processed foods, fried foods, preservatives and chemicals, and artificial sweeteners, flavors, and/or colors. Certain foods that will help the liver detox include beets, dandelion greens, artichoke tea (see the recipe in chapter sixteen), fresh lemon juice and pink Himalayan salt in filtered water, and you might also want to consider talking to your health practitioner about adding some other supplements or herbs to your diet such as milk thistle or alpha lipoic acid.

If you are wondering if your liver is needing a break, ask yourself the following questions:

1. Do you have elevated triglycerides or LDL cholesterol?

2. Do you have recurring pain or discomfort in the upper right corner of the abdomen, below the rib?

3. Have you had trouble with your gallbladder/gallstones, or do you have trouble digesting fatty foods?

4. Do you regularly take medications, recreational drugs, or synthetic hormones?

5. Do you work in an environment with a high exposure to chemicals, herbicides, or pesticides?

6. Do you regularly eat processed, packaged, or fast foods?

7. Do you rely mostly on sodas or sweetened beverages?

8. Do you drink more than two alcoholic beverages nightly or regularly wake up feeling hungover?

9. Are you overweight, especially in the midsection, or "top-heavy"?

10. Do you tend to see the negative side of every situation or have a short temper?

11. Do you have acne/rosacea, broken capillaries, or brown ("liver") spots on your skin?

12. Have you recently lost your appetite or had unexplained weight loss?

13. Do you have changes to your nails, including clubbing or a white "broken glass" appearance?

The more "yes" answers you gave to the questions above, the more TLC your liver probably needs, and the more gently and slowly you might want to support your liver to recover. Do not panic, and remember that the liver is very resilient. But realize that if there is more advanced liver disease, you will want the support of a professional. If you are concerned about your liver health, see your health practitioner to get some blood work done to find out if your liver enzymes are in balance. An ultrasound can identify if your liver has excess fat.

ARE OUR KIDS ACCUMULATING TOXIC FAT?

One of the most concerning things to me is the amount of toxins in the foods that we are feeding to our kids. Kids' bodies are more vulnerable to toxins, yet many of the foods marketed and designed for kids are some of the most toxic foods on the market. Lots of "kid foods" are loaded with sugars, flavorings, and chemicals that are specifically designed to be addictive! Kids are regularly consuming brightly colored candies and sports drinks; flavor-blasted chips that have MSG and trans fats and sodas sweetened with high fructose corn syrup. And by doing so, they are consuming obesogens, increasing the toxic load on their bodies, and raising the risk that they will become overweight and develop more serious health problems. Not surprisingly, we are seeing conditions like diabetes, heart disease, and fatty liver disease affecting an increasing number of young individuals today.

The Bottom Line

Although there is no way to avoid all toxins completely, there are several things that we can do to reduce our exposure. The first step is awareness—understanding where toxins are found and how to avoid them. The next step is to support the body to usher out toxins by supporting their elimination.

❧ 6 ❧

Put Out the Fire of Inflammation
"The Silent Killer"

*Inflammation leads to every one of the major chronic diseases of aging—
heart disease, cancer, diabetes, dementia, and more. It's also by far the
major contributor to obesity. Being fat is being inflamed—period!*

—DR. MARK HYMAN, *New York Times* best-selling author

We all have experienced inflammation—the bump on our head we
get when we bang it hard; the swelling and pain in our ankle that
happens if we twist it; the redness and irritation around a mosquito bite
or cut on our skin; or the swollen nose that comes with a cold or flu.
Inflammation is the body's response to an insult or injury. Part of the
healing process, ideally, inflammation is short-lived.

But sometimes the process can go awry. The signals go haywire, and
the inflammation can become chronic. Perhaps there is a chronic condition that is causing inflammation to stick around (such as an undiagnosed food intolerance, infection, etc.). Sometimes inflammation even
attacks the body's own cells as in autoimmune conditions. This can riddle
the body with *systemic* inflammation, which can affect our metabolism
as well as every organ, and lead to weight gain. This creates an environment ripe for disease. And because systemic inflammation may not be
accompanied by the typical symptoms, it can be left to silently progress.

Labeled "The Secret Killer" by *Time* magazine, inflammation is the
hallmark of many diseases. Chronic inflammation is a recognized factor in allergies, arthritis, heart disease, cancer, asthma, diabetes, eczema,
stroke, digestion problems (such as IBS and Crohn's), dementia, Alzheimer's, autoimmune diseases, and more. Yet, despite the fact that there is a

clear link between inflammation and many diseases, unfortunately, many of the symptoms of inflammation can go unnoticed. Just being overweight raises our inflammation because our adipose tissue secretes chemicals that promote inflammation in the body. Researchers have also found a link between insulin and inflammation, so keeping our blood sugar under control is very important for keeping inflammation in check.

"A Disease of Affluence"

According to Floyd Chilton, author of *Win the War Within*, "the more developed and industrialized the country, the more inflammatory disease there appears to be, which makes inflammation *a disease of affluence*." Studies show that people who emigrate to developed countries are more prone to develop inflammatory bowel disease. Perhaps this provides a clue to one of the main causes of the inflammation: a more highly processed diet.

You know the expression, "where there's smoke, there's fire." A fire can't just light itself; something has to start it. The same thing is true with inflammation. When inflammation is present in the body, we need to ask what set the fire in the first place.

Pain goes hand in hand with inflammation. And so people who are suffering from chronic pain should consider if chronic inflammation could be to blame. I personally used to suffer from chronic pain and inflammation, and because I did not have any clue that the root cause was undiagnosed food intolerances and excess sugar, I just bought ibuprofen in bulk. But taking lots of ibuprofen does nothing to deal with the root cause of the pain or inflammation. Taking a pill to deal with our inflammation is kind of like putting a fan in front of a fire: the smoke (symptoms) gets blown away, yet the fire (inflammation) underneath continues to burn. And as we know, when inflammation is allowed to continue, it can become systemic and develop into diseases.

Another downside to taking ibuprofen in bulk is the potential damage to the gut lining. Multiple studies have found a link between NSAID use and damage to the intestinal lining or leaky gut. So popping a lot of over-the-counter pain pills could be adding insult to injury.

Instead, look at the reason for the inflammation for a more permanent solution. This sometimes takes a little detective work because many different things can lead to chronic and uncontrolled inflammation. Here are some potential causes to consider:

- Undiagnosed food intolerances
- Chronic infections, such as periodontal disease, gut infections, or bacterial overgrowth
- Diets high in trans fats or damaged fat, polyunsaturated oils (such as soy, corn, and other high omega-6 fatty acids)
- Too many processed and packaged foods
- Consumption of too much sugar and high glycemic foods
- Poorly managed or excess stress
- Lack of exercise
- Being overweight, especially in the abdomen area (*This is both a cause and a symptom of systemic inflammation.*)
- Chronic exposure to chemicals/toxins

Some inflammation does not cause pain; it can have no symptoms at all. This *"silent inflammation"* is very dangerous because it can progress quietly and impact our brains and other organs.

Inflammation in the Brain

Because there are usually no symptoms of brain inflammation, we very likely will have no idea if our brain is suffering until it is too late. According to Dr. David Perlmutter in *Grain Brain,* "Researchers have known for some time that the cornerstone of all degenerative conditions, including brain disorders, is inflammation. And what they are finding is that gluten and a high carbohydrate diet are among the most prominent stimulators of inflammatory pathways in the brain." Dr. Perlmutter also points to elevated blood glucose as one of the main causes for inflammation and damage within the brain, which over time can lead to Alzheimer's, also referred to as "type 3 diabetes."

Inflammation and the Heart

According to Dr. Mark Houston, author of *What Your Doctor May Not Tell You About Heart Disease,* heart disease begins with damage to the endothelium, which can be caused by many different things including diets high in sugar, cigarette smoke, toxins, elevated blood pressure, and infections. Inflammation is the body's attempt to heal the damage to the endothelium. But unless the underlying reason for the inflammation is dealt with, it can become chronic and disease-promoting.

Knowing this, it should not be surprising that chronic and systemic inflammation are better predictors for a heart attack than high LDL cholesterol. According to a recent study out of UCLA, 75 percent of patients hospitalized for a heart attack had LDL cholesterol below 130 mg/dl, and 50 percent of patients had LDL below 100 mg/dl.

Autoimmune Diseases

A healthy immune system recognizes and attacks damaging substances, such as viruses, bacteria, fungi, or toxins. But sometimes, as in the case of autoimmune diseases, it becomes overactive and perceives the body's own tissues as a threat, attacking them. This can lead to inflammation over long periods of time. But the question remains, is an overactive autoimmune system a condition within itself or was it caused by something else, such as a food intolerance, chronic infection, or other insult? The answer may not come easily, but it is worth investigating to find the root cause and heal the body.

Inflammation and the Metabolism

Research shows that inflammation and insulin resistance appear to go hand in hand. And as we know from chapter one, when there is insulin resistance, the body is not effectively handling sugars and carbohydrates and storing more and more fat. This leads to a self-fulfilling cycle of metabolism meltdown: inflammation leads to insulin resistance, which causes the body to store more fat, those fat cells produce more inflammation, which leads to worse insulin problems, and so on.

The Wrong Fats

The kind of fats we are eating can either promote inflammation or help to reduce it. When it comes to fats, the body needs a balance of inflammation-lowering and inflammation-promoting fats.

- ꙮ **Omega-6 fatty acids,** which are high in linoleic acid and pro-inflammatory, include vegetable oils (such as corn, soy, cottonseed, sunflower), grain-fed beef, deep-fried foods, conventional eggs, and more. Processed foods are higher in omega-6s because they also contain the pro-inflammatory and damaged oils.

- **Omega-3 fatty acids** are inflammation-lowering and can be found in fatty fish, fish oils, grass-fed animal proteins, some seeds, nuts, and also algae.

Unfortunately, the Standard American Diet (SAD) is providing too many inflammatory omega-6 fats and is lacking in omega-3s. The ideal ratio of omega-3:omega-6 fats is about 1:3. But many American ratios are closer to 1:20.

Reducing your intake of omega-6 fats and increasing your intake of omega-3s are important for reducing inflammation. One way to boost omega-3s is to take chia seeds, which are a vegan form of ALA omega-3s. Because not everyone effectively converts the ALA form into the usable DHA and EPA, taking a high-quality fish oil is another good strategy to boost omega-3s in the blood. Ideally, you want a fish oil that offers a good dose of both the DHA and EPA forms and ensures a high quality and purity. Important for a healthy heart, brain function, a balanced mood, and disease prevention, omega-3s are one of the most important supplements that everyone should take for their overall health and disease prevention.

Studies have linked omega-3 intake to reduced body fat, reduced risk of depression and other mood disorders, and improved brain health. Research is also showing that omega-3s can offer powerful antiaging and anticancer benefits. Studies have shown that people with higher blood level concentrations of omega-3s have longer telomeres. Telomeres are found at the end of a strand of DNA and serve to protect the chromosome from deterioration. Longer telomeres are associated with longevity and antiaging. One note of caution with omega-3 fish oils: they can thin the blood. In the right amount this can be beneficial, but it is important to follow dosing recommendations on the package and/or consult your health practitioner about the right amount for you based on your individual needs, especially if you are already taking medications. . They should be stopped a few weeks before surgery too.

Trans Fats

Trans fats are known to promote inflammation by damaging the cells that line blood vessels, which is related to blockages in the arteries. They also can trigger free radicals, which can lead to inflammation and other diseases.

Sugar and Inflammation

Remember from chapter one that diets high in sugar also promote inflammation. When insulin is elevated, it can signal some inflammation messengers. So cutting back on sugar and refined carbs is an important step in reducing inflammation.

Gluten and Other Food Intolerances

Undiagnosed food intolerances can create chronic inflammation in the body and can lead to damage of the lining of the small intestine.

Steps to Take to Reduce Inflammation

1. Identify and remove foods that you are allergic or sensitive to (wheat/gluten and dairy are the top two offenders).

2. Identify and treat any chronic infections in the gut to reduce inflammation. This will also reduce allergic reactions and improve digestive issues.

3. Once infections have been removed, it is important to heal the digestive system and increase the healthy bacteria with probiotics (leaky gut can lead to chronic inflammation and pain).

4. Keep your pancreas from constantly sending out insulin. Avoid sweetened foods/drinks and foods with a high glycemic response (sugar, simple carbs, etc.).

5. Lose weight. Fat cells, especially those in the midsection, produce inflammatory molecules called cytokines, according to Dr. Peter Libby of Harvard, which can in turn produce chronic inflammation. For every 2.2 pounds lost, C-reactive protein was reduced by an average of 0.13 milligrams per liter, a report published in *Archives of Internal Medicine* found.

6. Reduce the amount of chemicals and toxins in your diet and environment, which can stimulate inflammation.

7. Take probiotics, because some research has linked certain unhealthy bacteria to inflammation and heart disease.

8. Reduce the foods that promote inflammation:

   ◆ Dairy/cow's milk

- Sugary foods and drinks and high glycemic foods
- Alcoholic beverages
- Omega-6 fatty acids (corn, soy, vegetable, cottonseed, and sunflower oils)
- Trans fatty acids

- Increase the foods that reduce inflammation:
  - Turmeric (called Nature's Advil)
  - Ginger
  - Green tea
  - Monounsaturated fats like olive and avocado
  - Omega-3 fats and foods:
    - Wild fatty fish such as salmon and sardines
    - High-quality fish oil supplements
    - Chia seeds, oil
    - Flaxseeds, oil
    - Tree nuts (such as almonds, walnuts)

Testing for Inflammation

If you are concerned about inflammation, you can ask your doctor for the high sensitivity C-reactive protein (hs-CRP) test, which measures inflammation in the body. Although not the only test available, the hs-CRP is recognized as a better indicator of heart disease risk than cholesterol levels. According to the American Heart Association, a C-reactive protein level of less than 1 mg/l indicates a low risk of cardiovascular disease, 1 to 3 mg/l indicates moderate risk, and greater than 3 mg/l equals high risk. Other tests that can help your doctor determine if you might have chronic inflammation include the cholesterol particle test and the homocysteine test.

The Bottom Line

Like so many things in the body, inflammation is about balance. It is needed for an acute healing crisis, but when it is systemic and chronic, it interferes with the metabolism and increases disease risk. When the body is under "attack" in this way, we can suffer from pain and swelling. Or it could be silently damaging our organs, as is often the case with the brain. Finding the root cause of and dealing with chronic inflammation are critical for a healthy metabolism and disease prevention. The good news is that optimizing blood sugar and digestion, removing foods we are intolerant to, and reducing stress all add up to lower inflammation.

<< 7 >>

Stop the Madness
Lower Stress, the "Switch that Turns on Disease"

Stress and anxiety are choices that we make, ways that we choose to process events. Each day we have hundreds of opportunities to shift our thoughts and align with the Source that intended us for lives of joy and peace.

—WAYNE DYER

Have you ever seen a hamster on his wheel? My daughter had two of them, and they would hop on that wheel and run like crazy! They ran like their lives depended on it, and they were going nowhere. Do you ever feel like those hamsters running on your proverbial wheel day in and day out, and wonder where it's getting you?

Most Americans are under way too much stress. Our culture is focused on working harder, faster, and constantly pushing ourselves. Each day we deal with traffic, deadlines, nonstop emails and texts, financial woes, and eating on the go. We are so focused on achieving, winning, getting ahead, and keeping up that the last thing on our minds is rest or relaxation. In fact, we feel guilty if we take time off or for ourselves. We admire people who work hard and can multitask. But even hamsters curl up into a little ball and sleep for hours on end when they are not zipping away on those wheels! We should take a cue from them, and start to realize the value of self-care.

Pushing through uncontrolled stress and not giving the body downtime to heal and recover can set us up for weight gain and even a health crisis of major proportions down the road. Stress is often considered a trigger that "turns on" disease. An Ohio University study discovered a "master gene" that is activated under stressful conditions called ATF3, which may be involved in the metastasis of cancer. Other studies have linked stress and negative emotional states to an increased risk of stroke, heart attack, and even brain shrinkage.

The Yin and Yang of Metabolism

According to the laws of nature and a fundamental concept in Chinese medicine, opposites are needed to balance each other out. Referred to as "yin and yang," there are examples all around us: the sun and the moon, female and male, light and dark, hot and cold, etc. There are many aspects of the metabolism that have yin and yang as well. One example is the body's stress response through the parasympathetic and sympathetic nervous systems. Each of these two systems is important for our internal balance, but when one is too dominant, it can set us up for a cascade of health problems.

Our autonomic nervous system (ANS) enables the brain to communicate with our organs, glands, peripheral nervous system, and some of our muscles. The ANS regulates important involuntary body functions including digestion, blood flow, heart rate, and respiration. There are two sides of our ANS:

- **The sympathetic nervous system (SNS)** is the "fight or flight" side of our ANS. When called into action, it uses energy to increase your heart rate, raise your blood pressure to increase blood flow, increase blood glucose to give you a boost, and dilate your pupils. It also turns off systems that are not needed, such as digestion, elimination, and reproduction.

- **The parasympathetic nervous system (PNS)** is the "rest and digest" side of our ANS. It is responsible for digestion, recovery, rest, and reproduction; it can also be called our "feed and breed" side. When the PNS is dominant, our blood pressure drops, pulse rate goes down, and our body can relax, recover, and digest. If we are stuck in a stress response, our bodies are not able to rest, digest, or recover.

Back in the days when we had to hunt and gather to live, there would be times when the fight or flight mechanism was lifesaving—such as when running from a predator. This kind of stress was usually short-lived, lasting just long enough to get out of harm's way. Once safe, the stress response would turn off, and the hunter-gatherer would go back to normal life (like that hamster when it gets off the wheel).

But in today's stressed-out lifestyles, our SNS is in gear all the time. This elevates our blood pressure and heart rate, stress hormones, and it suppresses our digestion and elimination. Stress can come in several different forms—emotional, mental, physical, including from our diet and environment. Emotional and mental stress can include anger, fear, sadness, loss, guilt, worry, depression, and anxiety. Physical stress can come from lack of sleep, chronic infection, a food intolerance, and even too much exercise. Diet and environmental stress can result from too much sugar and processed foods, a lack of sunshine, and exposure to chemicals. According to the American Institute of Stress, by far the biggest source of stress for adults is work.

Stress and that rush of adrenaline can also be addictive. This may be why many people like scary movies and roller coasters: they give us a temporary thrill. And like the hunter-gatherers, we generally return to a calm state after an exciting ride. But when we feel out of control and under constant stress, our body is not able to do the repair work it needs to do. We can eventually become lethargic, and our immune system can get worn out. And then we turn to foods and substances as our "crutches" to get us through the day.

Stress, Sugar, and Caffeine—Partners in Crime

The more stressed out and tired we get, the more sugar, caffeine, and carbs we tend to seek for quick energy. They are all partners in crime. If you are overdoing the sugar, caffeine is usually part of the roller-coaster equation. You end up running on that hamster wheel all day.

Can you relate to this scenario?

1. Alarm clock goes off at 6 a.m.

2. Hit the snooze button. Repeat as many times as possible and not lose job.

3. Glance over at the clock; it is 6:40 a.m.—eek, how'd that happen? Stress and panic kick in, which provide the adrenaline needed to jump out of bed.

4. Head down to the coffee machine. Stare at it dripping into the carafe while kids are screaming for breakfast and empty lunch boxes sit on the counter.

5. Coffee is ready, pour it. Load it up with sugar. Drink it. Now the day can begin.

6. Make breakfast, pack lunch boxes, get kids off to school.

7. Pour another coffee "for the road."

8. At work, energy starts to drag around 10 a.m., grab a muffin or a 100-calorie pack of cookies or a bar.

9. Lunchtime rolls around. Have a diet soda, sandwich, and a bag of chips.

10. Mid-afternoon slump rolls around. Time for a bag of pretzels and another diet soda or a coffee. Perhaps a few strolls by the candy dish in the office.

11. Dinnertime is here. No energy to cook, let's pick up takeout on the way home.

12. Back at home, pretty wired, yet also tired; a glass of wine might take the edge off. Another one with dinner too. And then, there is just a little left in the bottle. Why not finish it off? Dishes to wash? Too tired for that. Laundry to fold? There is the weekend for that.

13. Needing a little something sweet after dinner—maybe a little ice cream. Start with a spoonful, then a few more. Oops! Realize that you finished the whole pint.

14. Try to settle down to sleep, but despite being extremely tired, you are also oddly too wired to fall asleep. Pull out the iPad or turn on the TV to pass the time.

15. Finally fall asleep, only to wake up again around 3 or 4 a.m., and you are stressing about deadlines at work, so you can't seem to fall back asleep.

16. Alarm clock goes off at 6 a.m., and it all starts over again.

The above scenario was not too far from my life not too many years ago. I had a tenuous balance going with the caffeine. I had to drink enough coffee to start the engines, but not so much that I had a headache. *I didn't always find that perfect balance.* Looking back, I can't believe that I usually needed to hit the snooze button two to three times before I could drag myself out of bed! I was burning out my adrenals, my thyroid, and skirting the edge of autoimmune disease. I didn't even really think there was anything wrong with it at the time. I was like a car with no fuel left—just running on fumes. If you are in a cycle like this, it is important to lower stress levels, nourish the body, and support the adrenals (more about this in a moment).

Another Partner—Wine

After using caffeine, carbs, and sugar to get through our day, we might feel so tightly wound up we can't settle down in the evening without a drink or two. Wine and other alcoholic beverages take that "edge" off. And very much like the coffee, there can be a tenuous balance there. One glass is nice, but two might just help us relax more. Before you know it, the recycling container is filling up. Drinking also can negatively affect our sleep and puts added strain on our already overtaxed liver. Because alcohol increases urine output, it can cause dehydration, vitamin and mineral depletion, and make our blood "thicker," which can raise our risk of heart attack.

Let's look at how alcohol affects the body. Approximately 20 percent is absorbed in the stomach, with most of the remaining alcohol absorbed through the small intestine. The liver sends out enzymes to break down and metabolize it. Consuming more than the liver can metabolize causes acetaldehyde to accumulate in the blood and body tissues. The Latin root of intoxification is *intoxicare*, "to poison."

The good news? A moderate amount of wine does provide some anti-oxidants and stress relief. But this is a case where moderation really is key. Generally for women, the liver can only process about one ounce of alcohol (approximately one standard drink) on average in one hour; men can generally metabolize two drinks per hour. Regularly go beyond one drink per night for women, and two for men, and the benefits quickly get replaced with an increased risk of diseases, including cancer and heart disease. Taking a break from alcohol is an important way to support the liver and overall health.

If the idea of giving up alcohol for even one night does not seem possible to you, I recommend that you read *The Mood Cure* by Julia Ross. This wonderful text explains how amino acid supplementation can help people break free from alcohol, sugar cravings, depression, and much more.

HORMONE HIGHLIGHTS: THE STRESS HORMONES

Several hormones play a critical role in the body's stress response.

- **Cortisol.** A steroid hormone produced by the adrenal cortex, it is often referred to as the "stress hormone" because stress activates its secretion. During the normal course of any given day, our cortisol levels will fluctuate. Generally, our cortisol levels should be higher in the morning to give us a little "get up and go." Our cortisol should be lower in the evening and nighttime, in order to settle down to go and stay asleep. Cortisol is important because it can give us a quick burst of energy, heightened memory, lower sensitivity to pain, and improved awareness—all the kinds of things that would help if we were in danger and needed to escape or run away from a predator ("fight or flight"). But chronic stress in the modern world causes the adrenal glands to produce more cortisol, which can throw our rhythms off. For example, we can feel "tired but wired" at night if our cortisol levels are up. Then the next morning, they can be low, which is why we drag ourselves out of bed and need three cups of coffee to jump-start our engines. Prolonged high levels of cortisol can result in poor digestion, blood sugar and blood pressure issues, reduced immunity, bone density issues, and weight gain—especially in the midsection. When cortisol is elevated, so is the hormone insulin, which tells our body to store fat in our midsection. Having your cortisol levels checked is a good way to determine if stress is negatively affecting your health and weight.

- **Adrenaline.** This is also produced in your adrenal glands in response to a threat or stress. For example, if someone comes up to you and tries to rob you, your adrenaline would kick in so you could fight back or run away. But often our adrenal glands are pumping out too much adrenaline due to chronic stress in our lives.

- **Aldorsterone.** This hormone is responsible for maintaining the proper levels of sodium, potassium, and water in our cells, which in turn regulates our blood pressure and hydration levels. One sign of overworked adrenals can be light-headedness upon rising, indicating poor blood pressure regulation. Craving salt can be another sign that the body is overstressed and the adrenals need support. *See chapter nine for more information about sodium and hydration.*

- **Pregnenolone and the "Pregnenolone Steal."** When the body is under prolonged stress, cortisol levels can stay elevated for long periods of time. In order to keep pumping out more cortisol, the body has to:

  - Make more cholesterol to convert into cortisol. Cholesterol is the raw material from which all hormones are made, and so in times of stress, the body generates more cholesterol to keep up with the demand. This is how stress can elevate cholesterol levels.

  - Steals it. When the body is under chronic stress, it might not have or be able to make enough cholesterol to turn into cortisol. So then it will resort to stealing it from other hormones. This is called the "Pregnenolone Steal." Pregnenolone is the raw material from which estrogen and testosterone are made. When the body is under prolonged stress, it will co-opt the pregnenolone to produce cortisol, which means that the other hormones can get out of balance, potentially leading to low testosterone (low sex drive) and dangerous estrogen-dominant conditions.

Because repeatedly spiking cortisol also causes insulin to get elevated, out-of-control stress can also lead to insulin and leptin resistance. Stress can cause us to gain weight and be the switch that turns on disease.

So how do we get out of this scenario? It is not easy, and it does not happen overnight. Each of the ten keys in the Perfect

> Metabolism Plan can help you to line those metabolism domi-
> noes back up to put you well on your way to waking up and feel-
> ing refreshed, having the energy you need to get through the day,
> and feeling less wired and stressed at the end of the day.

The Adrenals

If we are in the early stages of being too stressed, often our cortisol levels
will be high, and we will be wired, short-tempered, and anxious. But
the longer our stress is out of control, the harder it gets for the adrenal
glands to keep up with the demand for pumping out cortisol. If we end
up with chronically low cortisol, we can have adrenal fatigue, character-
ized by crushing fatigue, low blood pressure, dehydration, depression,
and just difficulty getting through the day.

The adrenals are little grape-sized organs that sit above the kidneys,
and one of their primary jobs is to produce the hormones that prepare
the body for the fight or flight response. They are also involved in regulating the body's proper levels of water to sodium, blood pressure and
blood flow, blood sugar, and heart rate.

When we push through all the stress for too long, the adrenal glands
can get overworked. When they get depleted, they can no longer pump
out that adrenaline to keep us going. So we push harder with more coffee,
sugar, and carbs to make up the difference. That gets our motor running
for a few hours, but in the long run, it further depletes our adrenal glands.
When the adrenals get fatigued, their ability to produce sufficient cortisol
and other important hormones can be compromised. Rather than just
drinking more coffee and eating more sugar to carry on, the real answer
is dialing back the stress and supporting the adrenals.

The Sunshine Test for Adrenals

Are you one of those people who can't step outside for a moment without
your sunglasses? One symptom of adrenal fatigue is that the pupils may
not be properly dilating, which can make our eyes especially sensitive to
bright lights. This simple experiment can help to identify adrenal issues.

Adrenal Fatigue "Test": Go outside in the sunshine without your sunglasses (or into a dark room in front of a mirror with a flashlight). **Do not**

look directly at the sun (or the flashlight), but while facing perpendicular to the sun, open your eyes and allow some sunlight to *indirectly* enter your eyes. Do you struggle to keep them open? Is it really painful to try to open your eyes in the daylight without sunglasses? This can be an indication of adrenal issues. This test can also be part of the cure, because when sunlight is allowed to indirectly come into the occipital lobe, it can help to break up the calcifications of the pineal gland. Do this for 15 minutes a day—notice in a week or two if you are struggling less to open your eyes.

Other Symptoms of Adrenal Fatigue

Some further signs that the adrenals might be struggling are dizziness upon standing, feeling tired but wired in the evening before bed, foggy brain, dark circles under eyes, light-headedness, and stubborn weight gain inthe midsection. Finding some ways to consciously reduce and deal with stress is very important to our weight and our overall health. One of the best cures is also free of charge—sleep.

Sleep—The Magic Pill We Are Seeking?

How we feel during our waking hours has a lot to do with how well we are sleeping. Have you ever noticed that in addition to being tired, sluggish, and moody, you are also hungrier after a poor night's sleep? It's not your imagination: it's your hormones—specifically elevated ghrelin levels (the hormone that causes hunger spikes). When it is sleep deprived, our body loses the ability to regulate hormone levels. In fact, even one night of sleep deprivation can cause the body to show signs of insulin resistance, a major risk factor for diabetes. People who regularly sleep less than six hours a night are four and a half times more likely to develop insulin resistance. A recent study published in *Science Translational Medicine* showed that people who regularly get less than five and a half hours of sleep a night gain an average of ten pounds and suffer worsening glucose levels and increased risk of diabetes and metabolic syndrome. A recent study found that lack of sleep actually changed the composition of the fat cells, making them less sensitive to insulin. "Metabolically, lack of sleep aged fat cells about 20 years," said the study's senior author Matthew Brady, associate professor at the University of Chicago. He said that better sleep is a way to improve metabolic health.

At least 63 percent of women and 54 percent of men have trouble sleeping more than once per week according to the National Sleep Foundation

(NSF). A very important piece of our overall health, sleep is needed for the body to repair, recover, and regenerate. Our body cycles through different stages of rapid eye movement (REM) and non-rapid eye movement (NREM) sleep throughout the night, each providing something different. Interrupted sleep can cause us to miss out on the deeper sleep stages, which, according to the NSF, are the "most restorative" phases. During the third and fourth NREM stages, tissue growth and repair happen, energy is restored, and important hormones such as growth hormone are released. REM sleep is when we dream, which is important for our brain renewal and functioning.

Stress and lack of sleep go hand in hand and feed into each other. High stress levels can make us more wired and anxious, which can interfere with our ability to fall or stay sleep. Unfortunately, the less sleep we get, the less capable we are of handling stress. This can make settling down to a good night's sleep easier said than done. Here are some common sleep interrupters:

- **Alcohol.** Drinking alcohol can lead to a drop in blood sugar which can cause us to wake up in the middle of the night.

- **Restless leg syndrome.** Often an indication of a magnesium deficiency.

- **Sleep apnea/snoring.** Being overweight raises the risk for sleep apnea, so losing weight can help the situation. Sleep apnea also raises our risk of heart attack, consider seeing a specialist if you suffer from this.

- **Anxiety/stress.** When we are worried or anxious about something, it can be hard to fall or stay asleep. Doing something relaxing can reduce stress levels before bedtime. Consider reading, taking a bath, or listening to calm music.

- **Computers and other electronic devices.** Too much screen time can be stimulating, and the light they emit can confuse our sleep regulators. Turn all electronics off at least one hour before bedtime so you can settle down and get a good night's rest.

Some people find that some supplements can help support sleep and reduce anxiety, such as L-theanine, magnesium, or melatonin. Ask your doctor if these could be right for you and what the right dosage should be for your needs. You might also want to consider lowering the temperature in your bedroom, because a recent study published in the journal *Diabetes* found sleeping in a room cooled to sixty-six degrees to be associated with metabolic advantages including improved insulin sensitivity and higher levels of "brown fat," which is considered metabolically active or "good" fat. Raising the temperature of the room to eighty-five degrees reversed the benefits within four weeks.

Other Tips for Lowering Stress and Supporting the Adrenals

It is important to bring down our stress levels and do what we can for the adrenals. Some suggestions:

- ☙ **Gradually reduce your caffeine and stimulant intake.** Caffeine is a double-edged sword. Usually if our adrenals are fatigued, we rely on it to jump-start our day. But caffeine can end up depleting us over time, especially when we are taking it in all day long. Cutting back on caffeine in the long run will give you more energy. But do it gradually, because giving up caffeine too quickly or cold turkey can mean pounding headaches and crushing fatigue. Part two of this book will guide you on how to gradually cut back on the caffeine and offer some good alternatives to coffee.

- ☙ **Learn to say "no."** One of the reasons that we can find ourselves overwhelmed is because we tend to overcommit ourselves. If you are a "people pleaser," you probably say yes more than you really want to. Each time you agree to a new commitment, you put yourself lower on the priority list, so you have less time to take care of yourself. Obviously, there are things that you can't say no to, like work projects or other crucial commitments. But for other things, give yourself permission to say no, or "I am sorry, I am not able to do that right now" occasionally.

- ☙ **Get key nutrients.** Processed foods, sugar, and refined carbs can cause blood sugar instability and can negatively affect sleep cycles. Make sure you are eating a high-quality diet rich in plant-based foods that deliver vitamins, minerals, and electrolytes. Magnesium is particularly supportive of the adrenals, because it can calm the nervous system, promote relaxation and sleep, improve blood sugar regulation, and reduce anxiety. The B vitamins are also very important to replenish in times of stress or adrenal fatigue, so make sure you are getting plenty of high-quality proteins at each meal and consider supplementing with a high-quality B complex. Some adaptogenic herbs can be helpful in times of stress, such as ashwagandha and rhodiola. Adaptogens do exactly what their name implies: they help the body adapt to stress.

🌿 **Don't fear high-quality salt.** Americans are told to get the salt out of their diets, but a 2014 study published in the *New England Journal of Medicine* has revealed that the guidelines for sodium restriction may have been too stringent and that healthy individuals without blood pressure problems can safely consume between 3,000 and 6,000 milligrams daily. As with many things, quality is key when it comes to salt. I recommend tossing out processed pristine white table salt (sodium chloride), as the processing removes all the naturally occurring minerals. But unprocessed high-quality pink Himalayan or Celtic sea salt is another thing entirely. Mineral-rich crystal salt contains sodium that is bioavailable to the body and also delivers over eighty trace minerals important to overall health. High-quality mineral-rich salts often have a color—grayish for Celtic gray salt (traditionally used in fermentation) and pinkish for Himalayan. People who have adrenal issues generally have a higher need for *the good kind of salt*. When I am working hard or under excess stress, I like to add a pinch of pink Himalayan salt and a squeeze of fresh lemon to my water. And as long as you are using high-quality unprocessed salt, feel free to salt your foods to your taste.

🌿 **Don't go too long between meals**. I am generally not a fan of snacking all day long because that tends to spike blood sugar over and over. But when there is adrenal fatigue, it is very important to keep the body nourished and blood sugar stabilized. Going too long between meals can lead to blood sugar crashes as well as more nutrient deficiencies and neurotransmitter imbalances. Try to eat within the first hour of waking, and avoid going longer than four hours between eating. Do avoid the quick energy fixes of sugar, simple carbs, and caffeine, though, and instead follow the Rule of Three, which helps to stabilize blood sugar by having one or more of the following each time you eat: a healthy fat, protein, and/or fiber.

- **Don't overexercise.** Exercise is a form of physical stress on the body, especially long bouts of cardio. When the adrenals are compromised, it is important to not work out to excess, because that can just further deplete the adrenals. Nourishing exercise like yoga and walking is beneficial. When you do not feel like you have enough energy to exercise, listen to your body and let it rest. *Chapter ten goes into more depth on exercise.*

- **Identify food intolerances or gut infections.** Eating foods that we are intolerant to or having a hidden gut infection can be a source of chronic stress on the body which can lead to adrenal issues. Infections and intolerances create a cascade of symptoms ranging from poor absorption, digestion issues, poor nutrient absorption, thyroid issues, and more.

- **Laugh.** There are multiple studies that show that laughter is bona fide medicine, and it can go a long way in helping to reduce stress levels. Watch a funny movie or TV show, or get together with people who make you laugh.

Meditation

Shown to lower blood pressure, slow the heart rate, reduce cortisol levels, and even reduce inflammation in the body, meditation can be a powerful tool in combating stress and creating life transformation. It helps to build mindfulness and can even literally rewire your brain!

You might be thinking that meditation is too "out there" for you, but some of the world's most successful people, including Oprah Winfrey and Bill Ford, credit much of their success to regular meditation.

Maybe it is the idea of sitting still and doing nothing for twenty minutes that sounds impossible. If the thought of trying to fit meditation in to an already overscheduled day adds to your stress levels, let me introduce you to Dina Proctor, the creator of the 3x3 method of meditation. It turns out that as little as three minutes can make a difference!

Dina Proctor, author of the book *Madly Chasing Peace, How I Went from Hell to Happiness in 9 Minutes a Day,* came up with the 3x3 method of meditation in which she suggests that we meditate for just three minutes, three times a day. Her book is a powerful story about how meditation basically saved her and eventually transformed her life, in just nine minutes a day!

I also like to do what I call "walking meditation." I grab the leash and hit the hills around my home with my dog, and that is how I clear my head. Find ways that work for you to bring some calmness into your life—your metabolism and health will thank you.

What Is Your *Soul Food?*

Another important piece of our stress puzzle that is often missing is *soul food.* I am not talking about the fried chicken and okra kind of soul food. This *soul food* is something that we *experience* or *feel,* something that we enjoy doing that feeds our soul. Soul food can be almost anything that fills your heart and soul. It could be practicing yoga or crocheting. It can come from loving relationships or a fulfilling career. Maybe you have found a cause that you believe in, and your heart fills up when you donate your time to it. Maybe it is as simple as getting together with friends or family for an occasional walk in the park or game of cards. Maybe it is walking the dog and listening to music. It could be writing in a journal or drawing. The list of things that can feed our soul is endless—and also very personal. But despite that, too many of us are not getting any soul food at all. In fact, we might even feel guilty if we take the time to do something *just for ourselves.* Often, it is the most thoughtful, giving, and kind people who save the least amount of time for something they enjoy. And because of that, "people pleasers" often find themselves with an extra fifteen pounds around the waist and no time or energy left to do anything about it.

> ❧ Ask yourself: When was the last time you did something that *just you* love to do? That fills your heart and soul? That brings you joy? That relaxes you or makes you smile? For many of us, it may have been so long that we don't even really know what our soul

food is anymore! Now is the time to figure it out and even schedule it into your day. If you are someone who feels guilty taking time for yourself, just remind yourself that you are a better friend/mom/sister/employee when you fit in your own soul food.

The Bottom Line

We can only run on those hamster wheels for so long; our bodies eventually are going to reach a breaking point. Chronic stress can be the "switch" that lowers our immune systems, turns on disease, and slows down our metabolism. High levels of stress cause accelerated aging. According to Dr. Perricone, "massive amounts of cortisol can destroy the immune system, shrink the brain and other vital organs, decrease muscle mass, and cause thinning of the skin." Finding ways to reduce stress and improve sleep is important if we want to reset our metabolism, prevent the physical signs of aging, and lower our risk for disease.

❧ 8 ❧

Ditch the Convenience Foods
Your Body Needs Nutrients!

If it's a plant, eat it. If it was made in a plant, don't.

—MICHAEL POLLAN, RULE 19 FROM *FOOD RULES*

In our busy, over-scheduled lives, it is easy to rely on "convenience foods." But far too many of these are highly processed, calorie-dense, and nutrient-deficient. In fact, a diet high in the sugar, salt, and bad fats found in convenience foods causes the body to use up important nutrients in order to process them! So instead of being nourishing, I think of many packaged and fast foods as "robbing" the body. Our bodies work really hard all day long. We need nourishment for energy, growth, repair, digestion, and so much more. If we have nutrient deficiencies, it could lead to fatigue, fogginess, a sluggish metabolism, and worse—an increased risk of diseases.

When we take a closer look at all the potential health problems that can stack up from a highly processed diet, *most convenience foods really are not so convenient.*

When buying foods that come in a package or box, it is important to pay attention: read labels and be aware of which ingredients are nutritious—and which ones are not! There are a number of great companies that put high-quality ingredients into their products. I call those upgraded convenience options!

Eat Real Food!

One of the best ways to improve our metabolism and health is to kick all processed and packaged foods to the curb and simply eat more ***real food!***

How do you know if a food is *real?*

Real foods are clean, fresh, and nutrient-dense:

- ❧ **Clean** foods are free from chemicals, additives, GMOs, hormones, antibiotics, heavy metals, and other toxins.

- ❧ **Fresh** foods are unrefined and will eventually go bad. You will find fresh foods by shopping around the perimeter of the store. Foods with a long shelf life are not fresh. They tend to be in boxes, bags, etc. A long shelf life is good for the manufacturer's profits but not for our bodies.

- ❧ **Nutrient-dense** foods are rich in the micro- and macronutrients that the body needs. How do you know if your food is nutrient-dense? This chapter will cover some key nutrients that your body needs, why we can be deficient, and where to get them.

Let's take a closer look at some of the key nutrients that drive our metabolism. They are broken down into the macronutrients and the micronutrients.

The Macronutrients

Food macronutrients are the "major building blocks" that the body needs every day—proteins, carbohydrates, and fats. Because chapter two covered fats and chapter six discussed the importance of balancing the essential fatty acids, I will focus on protein and carbohydrates here.

Proteins: Choose Grass-Fed, Free-Range, Organic "Clean Proteins"

About 20 percent of our body weight is composed of proteins. Often referred to as the body's primary "building blocks," dietary proteins are crucial for the formation of muscle tissue, hormones, neurotransmitters, nerves, and organs. Protein also plays a role in cellular hydration and heart health by working to maintain the balance of sodium to potassium in cells. Eating protein also helps to stabilize the blood sugar.

Proteins are composed of chains of amino acids. The nine "essential amino acids" must come from foods because the body cannot manufacture them. Other amino acids, the human body can manufacture, some of which are called nonessential (the body can make them) or conditionally essential (the body can make them if other cofactors are present). Proteins that contain all the essential amino acids are considered complete (such as animal proteins). If they are missing essential amino acids, they are incomplete (most plant proteins). To make complete proteins out of incomplete ones, you need to know how to properly combine plant-based foods (such as eating beans and rice together). *This is why vegans and vegetarians need to be educated and disciplined about how to properly combine incomplete proteins and can often benefit from supplements to prevent amino acid deficiencies.*

Probably one of the most important things to keep in mind with proteins is quality, quality, quality. Remember from the chapter on toxins that we eat what the animal ate, so it is important to choose free-range, organic animal proteins. Not only do organic grass-fed proteins contain higher levels of omega-3 fats, vitamins, and minerals; they also do not contain any hormones, steroids, or antibiotics. Another consideration is to avoid burning or charring meats because cooking at very high heats can damage even the most stable of fats to generate toxins.

How much protein do we need? It depends on each body and activity level. Those of us who are more active will need more than those who are less active. Most people generally get sufficient protein. But if you are a heavy carbohydrate eater, replacing some of your carbohydrates with protein can benefit the metabolism. A study published in the *American Journal of Clinical Nutrition* found that increasing protein intake from 15 to 30 percent of the diet resulted in decreased appetite and weight loss. Picture one-quarter to one-third of your plate having protein (incomplete or complete). It is also possible to consume too much protein, which can often occur from taking too many protein supplements like protein powders and bars. Excess protein will just be converted and stored as adipose tissue and can be acidifying to the body.

Good complete protein choices are grass-fed organic beef, liver, lamb, pork, chicken, wild fish, and, for those who can tolerate them, eggs and raw dairy. There are some complete plant-based proteins including quinoa, hemp, and chia seeds. Incomplete proteins can be eaten together to make complete ones: nuts, legumes, rice, and grains (preferably nongluten).

Carbohydrates: Go for "Slow Carbs"

Carbohydrates are chains of sugars. These chains can be simple or complex. In order for carbohydrates to be converted into energy, they are broken down into individual sugar molecules.

One way to think about carbs is whether they are digested fast or slow. Remember in chapter one where we discussed the glycemic index? Simple carbohydrate chains such as sugar, candy, soda, processed grains, etc., are converted into sugars quickly. These can be considered high glycemic or "fast carbs." After intense exercise, you might need a fast carb to replenish depleted sugars and glycogen, but generally eating a lot of fast carbs over time can lead to insulin problems and other related health issues (see chapter one).

If a food takes longer to be converted into sugar, then it is considered a complex "slow carb." Slow carbs do not spike the blood sugar as high or as fast. Slow carbs include most non-starchy vegetables, fiber-rich (ideally nongluten) whole grains, seeds, nuts, and low glycemic starchy vegetables.

Each person needs a different amount of carbohydrates in their diet depending on their activity level and metabolic factors like insulin sensitivity. Less active people will need fewer carbohydrates than their more active counterparts. Emphasize your intake of slow carbs (especially plant based), and try to avoid nutrient-deficient processed carbs.

Plants Can Save Your Life!

One of the very best things we can do for our overall health is to simply eat more plant-based foods, especially non-starchy vegetables. Eating more plant-based foods can make us feel fuller, give us more energy, provide the body with nutrients, and even potentially save our lives! Numerous studies have shown that the more plant-based foods we eat (especially vegetables), the lower our risk of diseases such as cancer and cardiovascular disease—and even death. The Harvard Nurses' Health Study found that a higher intake of fruit and vegetables was associated with reduced risk of heart attack. Those who averaged eight or more servings of fruits and vegetables had a 30 percent lower risk of heart attack or stroke compared to those who ate less than 1.5 servings daily. And another study found that having seven or more servings of fruits and vegetables was associated with a 42 percent reduced risk of death (compared to those who ate less than one serving). It all almost sounds too good to be true! So why don't we eat more plant-based foods?

Some people avoid plant-based foods because they have trouble digesting them and end up with bloating and gas. There are several ways to deal with this. First, you will want to gradually increase your intake of plant-based and high-fiber foods to allow your digestive system to adjust. Underlying gut inflammation or bacterial imbalances could be leading to digestive distress. By removing common food intolerances and healing the gut, people might find that they can start to tolerate more fiber-rich foods. Cooking vegetables can make them easier on the digestion. Ideally, you will want to work toward about 50 percent of your plant-based foods to be raw. But feel free to lightly cook more (even all) of your vegetables if you need to for your digestion, especially initially—just do not cook them so much that they are limp, gray, and lifeless. In fact, some vegetables are actually better for us cooked. The lycopene in tomatoes, for instance, is significantly more powerful and bioavailable when cooked. Mushrooms are better for us cooked. The cruciferous vegetables like cabbage, broccoli, and brussels sprouts are more easily digestible when cooked, and cooking also helps to reduce goitrogens, which can be thyroid interrupters.

Did you know that according to the Harvard School of Public Health, an average person eating a 2,000-calorie diet should eat **nine servings (four and a half cups) of plant-based foods each day?** Unfortunately, the average American eats less than three total servings of fruits and vegetables each day, and many people get even fewer. One-quarter of the population gets less than one serving of vegetables a day, and over one-third gets less than one daily serving of fruit. If you took french fried potatoes out of the equation, it would probably be lower than that (french fries should not count)!

A visual goal to set is to try to fill one-third to one-half your plate with plant-based foods at each meal—the majority of which should be non-starchy vegetables. Vegetables are rich in antioxidants, low glycemic, reduce inflammation, and improve energy. They also provide a lot of fiber, which helps boost digestion and fills you up! Remember to eat your veggies with some fat—to help absorb your fat-soluble vitamins and keep you satisfied longer. So a little grass-fed butter on your broccoli is good!

Eat a Rainbow!

One of my favorite things to teach kids about nutrition is to "*eat a rainbow*," but it applies to everyone! Each different color of the rainbow tells us something about the kind of nutrients in that plant food. So when we choose a rainbow of colors, we are getting a wider variety of benefits to the body. Antioxidants not only give foods their vibrant colors, but they also protect cells from oxidation, encourage cell growth, fight inflammation, and sweep up free radicals to prevent oxidation and cell dysfunction. We can see oxidation in action when a sliced apple turns brown. But a little squeeze of lemon juice delivers antioxidants that can prevent the oxidation. Oxidative stress appears to be an important part of many human diseases and is linked to cancer, diabetes, heart disease, macular degeneration as well as the physical signs of aging.

Superfoods

There is a special category of highly nutrient-dense foods called *superfoods*! Superfoods are basically what their name claims: super nutritious, naturally low in sugar, and offering disease-prevention benefits! Some can be more exotic (dragon fruit, camu camu berries, bee pollen), while others are pretty common (spinach, blueberries, sweet potatoes). Even just adding in a few of these foods to our daily routine can have a huge impact on our metabolism, energy, disease prevention, and overall health.

Some of my favorite superfoods:

- **Chia seeds.** One of my favorite superfoods of all time—high in omega-3s, protein, calcium, iron, and a unique hydrophilic fiber—chia seeds are the main reason that I decided to become a nutritionist. I could not believe that one little seed could do so much to improve my energy, digestion, mood, skin, hydration, and more. I take two tablespoons of well-hydrated chia seeds every day.

- **Hemp seeds.** A vegetarian source of protein, omega-3s, fiber, and antioxidants, hemp seeds are versatile and have a mild nutty taste. Hemp is rich in an omega-6 called gamma-linolenic acid, which unlike other omega-6s is not pro-inflammatory, but instead is known to support healthy hormone balance.

- **Avocado.** Full of healthy monounsaturated fats that help to reduce our inflammation, absorb fat-soluble vitamins, and improve blood sugar control, avocados also are a surprisingly high-fiber food. A good source of carotenoids, vitamin K, vitamins B5 and B6, vitamin C, folate, and potassium, avocados promote bone and heart health. Adding avocados to smoothies can make them light and fluffy, boost the fiber, and vitamin content, and help to keep you satisfied longer.

- **Dragon fruit.** Also known as pitaya, this fascinating and exotic fruit is both beautiful and nutritious. It is a naturally low-sugar food and contains vitamin C, fiber, antioxidants, and omega-3s from the plethora of seeds in the flesh. The color of the dragon fruit flesh can be pale white or vivid pink, depending on where it is grown. The dark-pink color is believed to have more nutrients and antioxidants. I like to use dragon fruit in my smoothies. You can buy them in frozen smoothie packs from a company called Pitaya Plus.

- **Raw cacao.** With an oxygen radical absorbance capacity (ORAC) score of 95,500 per 100 grams, cacao is a superpower for preventing free radical damage. It is also one of the best-known food sources of magnesium, which is a very important nutrient that most people are deficient in. Cacao is also rich in potassium, iron, polyphenols, flavanols, theobromine, and proanthocyanidins. Cacao offers a long list of health benefits including reducing the risk of heart attack and stroke, lowering blood pressure, boosting mood and brain function, lowering stress, relaxing muscles, boosting our skin's internal SPF, and much more. A recent *Journal of Physiology* study suggests that cacao may help bolster exercise endurance. Look for raw cacao, which means it has not been heated, so more of the nutrients are preserved.

- **Sweet potatoes.** Despite their naturally sweet taste, sweet potatoes have a lower glycemic index than regular potatoes, which means they can be absorbed and used gradually, preventing the blood sugar from spiking and crashing. Sweet potatoes have been shown to improve blood sugar, even in type 2 diabetics.

One of the best sources of beta-carotene, sweet potatoes raise our blood levels of vitamin A, which is a fat-soluble vitamin and best absorbed when eaten with some dietary fat, so don't be afraid to put a little grass-fed butter on them! Sweet potatoes are a good carbohydrate source for athletes and also helpful in preventing inflammation, which aids in recovery.

- **Blueberries.** Rich in fiber, minerals, and the vitamins A, C, E and K, fresh blueberries are lower on the glycemic index than many fruits and also offer a good dose of fiber—both of which are helpful in managing blood sugar. A cup of blueberries has about 25 percent of the RDA of vitamin C. When given the choice between wild or cultivated berries, choose the wild. Despite being smaller than the cultivated kind, they contain more anthocyanins, which are known for their antiaging properties.

- **Dark leafy greens like kale and spinach.** High in nutrients like vitamin K, magnesium, vitamin C, calcium, folate, zinc, and iron, dark leafy greens are good for the health of our eyes, bones, heart, and immunity.

- **Almonds.** A good source of vitamin E, magnesium, potassium, manganese, copper, riboflavin, monounsaturated fats, and protein, almonds are nutritional powerhouses. A small handful of almonds a few times a week can be helpful in lowering cholesterol and preventing heart disease. Almonds are beneficial for the nervous system and useful for muscle recovery.

- **Coconut oil.** One of the best metabolism-boosting fats. I like to add one teaspoon to my morning cup of tea (or coffee if I am not eliminating it). See chapter two for more info about coconut oil.

- **Green tea.** A wonderful substitute for coffee, green tea has powerful compounds called polyphenols. One polyphenol in green tea is EGCG (epigallocatechin-3-gallate), which may reduce the risk of breast cancer. One study of Asian-American women found that those who drank more green tea were less likely to develop breast cancer. Another compound in green tea is the amino acid L-theanine, which is shown to reduce heart rate and promote focus and attention, while reducing anxiety levels and promoting calmness. Other benefits of drinking green tea instead of coffee are that it is less acidic and has lower caffeine levels.

Micronutrients in Food: Some Key Vitamins and Minerals

Micronutrients are vitamins, minerals, and trace minerals needed for cellular functions. Highlighted below are those that are very important to a healthy metabolism, as well as their key functions and some common food sources.

B Vitamins

The B vitamins are critical for a healthy metabolism, to support detoxification, and to convert our food into energy. Often referred to as *"the stress vitamins,"* B vitamins are water soluble, so they are not stored in the body for long, and stress accelerates their excretion. They are important for energy, mood, sleep, nerve function, digestion, heart health, and more.

- **Vitamin B12** (cobalamin) is needed for the metabolism of fats and amino acids, and is important for energy, mood, memory, and focus. A B12 deficiency can cause anemia, memory and focus issues, and nerve damage. It also might play a role in depression. Because B12 is naturally only available in animal proteins, it is very common for vegans to be deficient unless they are supplementing. Having inadequate levels of stomach acid or digestive disorders can also cause a B12 deficiency. Food sources include sardines, cod, tuna, chicken, beef, lamb, salmon, and dairy.

- **Vitamin B6** (pyridoxine) is important for the metabolism of carbohydrates, sleep, controlling inflammation, gallbladder health, and hormone balance. B6 is also very important for the production of neurotransmitters, which are important brain chemicals. A B6 deficiency can lead to PMS, low levels of serotonin or other neurotransmitters, and gallbladder trouble. Taking birth control pills and hormone replacement depletes B6. Food sources include tuna, turkey, chicken, salmon, beef, sweet potatoes, beans, and bananas.

- **B9** (folic acid/folate) is important for cellular growth and regeneration, as well as the prevention of colon cancer, heart disease and stroke, and birth defects. Folic acid deficiencies can show up as elevated homocysteine, which can damage blood vessels and raise the risk of heart disease. This can happen despite supplementation if someone has problems with methylation (conversion of the B vitamins). Folate is the natural form of B9 found in foods, whereas folic acid is the synthetic supplement form. Not everyone is able to convert folic acid to it's useable form. So it is a good idea to eat foods rich in folate. And if you do supplement, to use methyl-folate, which is more bio-available. Foods rich in folate include spinach, broccoli, asparagus, lentils, and several other legumes. A study conducted in the Netherlands found that taking the active methyl form of folic acid restored endothelial function in those with familial hypercholesterolemia.

- **B1** (thiamine) is needed for carbohydrate metabolism and is an important key to digestive health because it supports the production of hydrochloric acid in the stomach. Deficiencies can result in low stomach acid and fatigue and can hamper detoxification pathways of the liver. Food sources include organ meats, fish, pork, eggs, and dairy.

- **B3** (niacin) is important for the metabolism of sugars and the production of hormones, including the stress hormones. There is some evidence that niacin can help fight candida overgrowth and aid in lowering cholesterol levels. Care should be taken when supplementing with niacin, however, because higher doses or taking it over a long period could be toxic to the liver (for this reason long-acting niacin should be avoided). Niacin can also cause increased blood flow to the cheeks, causing a "niacin flush." Food sources include sardines, tuna, chicken, lamb, shrimp, and turkey.

- **B2** (riboflavin) is kind of like a starter engine for activating the B vitamins and glutathione, which is an important antioxidant for the liver. B2 is also needed for proper functioning of the red blood cells. Deficiencies could lead to migraine headaches. Food sources include liver, spinach, yogurt, almonds, mushrooms, and eggs.

🌀 **B5** (pantothenic acid) is important for the metabolism of all the macronutrients. B5 is also important for healthy skin and the adrenals, blood pressure and the thyroid. Food sources include mushrooms, cauliflower, avocados, lentils, sweet potatoes, and turkey.

Many people will benefit from taking a B complex supplement during this program and beyond. I recommend choosing a high-quality B complex with the methylcobalamin form of B12 (not the cyanocobalamin form) and the active methyl form of folic acid (methylfolate) because many people do not effectively convert the other forms.

Vitamin C

Vitamin C is an important antioxidant that supports detoxification, immune health, bone formation, wound healing, iron absorption, neurotransmitter synthesis, and skin health. Water soluble, vitamin C is not stored, so it must be regularly consumed. During times of stress, the body needs more to support the adrenals. Food sources of vitamin C are cabbage, peppers, citrus fruits, strawberries and other berries, broccoli, and tomatoes. I prefer to obtain vitamin C from food sources, because high doses of synthetic vitamin C (ascorbic acid) can damage the gut lining and upset the delicate balance of gut bacteria. You can find whole food vitamin C supplements made out of camu camu or acerola cherry.

Vitamin A

A key player in our immune system health, vitamin A is a fat-soluble vitamin that is important for healthy skin, eyes, reproduction, and cellular repair. It also has inflammation-lowering properties and supports free radical repair. Animal sources deliver the retinoid form of vitamin A and include liver, beef, cod liver oil, salmon, shrimp, sardines, eggs, and grass-fed butter. The vitamin A that is obtained from plants like sweet potatoes, carrots, pumpkin, spinach, and squash is the carotenoid form, which needs to be converted into the active retinoid form. Ideally, both forms of vitamin A should be obtained from the daily diet.

Because excesses of the retinol form of vitamin A are not readily excreted like the water-soluble vitamins, care should be taken when supplementing to prevent excess accumulation. Vitamin A toxicity is rare in the average person, but retinol supplementation may not be appropriate for those with liver disease, fat malabsorption, lung cancer, a bleeding disorder, or other conditions such as heavy alcohol use.

Vitamin D

Not really a vitamin but a fat-soluble prehormone, vitamin D is referred to as the "sunshine vitamin" because the sun is the best source. Vitamin D levels can fluctuate throughout the year, with levels typically dropping the most in the fall/winter months. Not surprisingly after years of slathering on sunscreen, a high percentage of people are now deficient in vitamin D.

I cannot emphasize the importance of this nutrient enough: having optimal levels of vitamin D could *literally save your life*! According to UCSD professor and researcher Cedric Garland, maintaining a vitamin D level between 40 and 60 ng/ml could prevent 58,000 new cases of breast cancer and 49,000 colorectal cancers each year. Insufficient levels of vitamin D also raise our risk of fractures and osteoporosis, inflammation, leaky gut, MRSA infections, heart disease, and breast cancer. Several studies have also found a link between low vitamin D status and poor blood sugar control and obesity. A 2012 University of Copenhagen study found a link between low vitamin D and heart disease.

According to the *New England Journal of Medicine*, a vitamin D deficiency is defined as circulating levels of 25-hydroxyvitamin D less than 32 ng/ml. Many studies suggest that optimal blood serum levels are around 50 ng/ml. How do you know if you have low vitamin D? You may not have any symptoms at all, or you might suffer from unexplained muscle or bone aches, weakness and pains, and/or depression. Sometimes, a bone fracture will alert someone to low vitamin D levels.

Food sources are limited and include fortified foods like pasteurized milk (generally fortified with D2, which is less effective than D3). Other food sources are salmon, sardines, and mushrooms (that have been exposed to the sun).

Most adults can benefit from 2,000 IU of vitamin D daily; some might need more depending on their blood levels. According to the Vitamin D Council, "In order to receive the most health benefit from increased levels of vitamin D, the proper cofactors must be present in the body including: vitamin K, vitamin A, zinc and boron, and magnesium." Magnesium is especially important for absorption, so I recommend that people take their vitamin D with their magnesium supplement. Certain medications, a low-fat diet, or a genetic defect for vitamin D conversion can also affect vitamin D absorption; check with your doctor or pharmacist if you are taking vitamin D but your levels are not going up or if you have questions. Vitamin D levels can fluctuate, so make sure to get your levels tested at least once yearly.

Magnesium

Referred to as the "relaxation mineral," it is estimated that 70 percent of the population may be deficient in magnesium, which is required for over 300 enzymatic reactions, including the synthesis of fat, protein, and nucleic acids, muscular contraction and relaxation, nerve health, bone building, and heart health.

Magnesium improves blood flow and plays a key role in serotonin production, protein building, and the metabolism of adenosine triphosphate (ATP). Magnesium helps rid the body of toxins and acid residues and is needed for the synthesis of vitamin D and absorption of calcium. An important mineral for our heart health, magnesium is also emerging as a player in cancer prevention. A study from Sweden reported that women with the highest magnesium intake had a 40 percent lower risk of developing cancer than those with the lowest intake of the mineral.

Low magnesium levels could be more of a factor than we all realize when it comes to a sluggish metabolism. Magnesium has been found in studies to improve insulin sensitivity, support healthy glucose metabolism, and stimulate the release of the fat-burning hormone adiponectin.

Food sources of magnesium include leafy greens, seeds (like pumpkin), avocados, broccoli, and beans. But perhaps the best (and most delicious) way to get magnesium is from raw cacao—the main ingredient in dark chocolate (see chapter sixteen for yummy raw cacao recipes).

Some symptoms of low magnesium levels are muscle twitches, muscle cramps, Leichtling irritability, constipation, migraine headaches, insomnia, chronic fatigue syndrome, kidney stones, and heart disease.

Calcium

Calcium is well-known for its role in healthy bones and teeth. But it also plays a part in the activation and secretion of enzymes and hormones, nerve impulses, and blood clotting. In order for calcium to get into the bones and teeth, it needs to have the necessary cofactors and be a form of calcium that is well-absorbed. Cheap, poorly absorbed forms of calcium supplements without the key cofactors can end up in places where it is not wanted, such as creating calcifications of the arteries and kidneys. So ideally calcium supplements should be highly absorbable forms of calcium (like algae based) and contain the necessary cofactors in the right proportion for absorption, including vitamin K, vitamin D, magnesium, and trace minerals. Food sources include sardines, sesame seeds, dairy products, broccoli, tofu, leafy greens, and salmon.

Should I Use Supplements?

I am a big proponent of obtaining the *majority* of our nutrients from foods, because they contain a synergistic combination of vitamins, minerals, and phytochemicals—all of which enhance the absorption and utilization by the body. Antioxidants in foods help fight free radical damage, reduce inflammation, and prevent illness and disease.

Those who consume very few plant-based foods, are vegan, follow a limited diet, or eat a highly processed diet will benefit from filling in dietary gaps with some high-quality supplements. But even people who eat a high-quality diet rich in plant-based foods could have deficiencies for any of the following reasons:

- **Poor soil quality.** Soils are increasingly becoming depleted, so much of our food is becoming more depleted as well. Buying organic certainly helps, as organic food tends to be grown in better soil, and your body won't have to deal with all the pesticides either.

- **Low stomach acid.** If you have low stomach acid, you might not be effectively breaking down and absorbing the nutrients you take in. Low stomach acid becomes even more prevalent as we age. Improving stomach acid with Bragg Lemonade or a digestive enzyme can help with this.

- **Digestive trouble.** Food allergies and intolerances, bacterial overgrowth, or other gut issues can also inhibit absorption and utilization of nutrients. Removing food intolerances and correcting digestive issues can help with this. But supplementation can be good for people avoiding food groups to ensure all key nutrients are getting delivered.

- **Antinutrients.** Some compounds in foods prevent the body from absorbing nutrients; these are called antinutrients. For example, phytic acids in grains, nuts, and soy can bind to and prevent the uptake of important minerals like zinc and magnesium. Soaking, sprouting, and fermenting can reduce or eliminate phytic acids to make the nutrient more bioavailable to the body. Lectins such as wheat germ agglutinin are another kind of antinutrient.

- **Missing key cofactors.** Certain nutrients need cofactors to be absorbed, such as calcium and fat-soluble vitamins. If you are missing key cofactors for absorption, you might not be absorbing all your nutrients.

- **Prescription medications or alcohol abuse.** Taking certain prescription medications or heavy alcohol use can lead to vitamin, mineral, and hormone deficiencies. Author Suzy Cohen, RPh, wrote *Drug Muggers* to help people understand which medications deplete nutrients and how to replenish them.

- **Genetic defects.** Having a genetic defect—such as a methylation defect—can lead to a reduced ability to convert certain nutrients into their usable form. Genetic testing may be able to identify a defect that could compromise your ability to convert nutrients. NeuroScience, Inc., offers several genetic testing options.

How Can I Tell If I Have Deficiencies?

There may or may not be symptoms at all, but nutrient deficiencies can show up in many different ways ranging from fatigue, weight gain, migraine headaches, neurological symptoms, focus issues, cravings, and much more. For those who want to know if they have specific nutrient deficiencies, you can get a test called the SpectraCell Micronutrient test, which measures functional levels of thirty-five nutritional components including vitamins, antioxidants, minerals, and amino acids in the white blood cells.

Choosing Supplements

I always caution people against buying the cheapest supplement because poor-quality supplements tend to be poorly absorbed, and worse, they might even do harm. For example, cheap calcium supplements that are missing the key cofactors for absorption into the bone can cause the calcium to migrate to where it should not go, potentially causing calcifications of the arteries and increasing the risk of heart disease.

The Bottom Line

A highly processed and nutrient-deficient diet can add up to increased hunger, cravings, low energy, mood swings, and weight imbalances. The body needs key nutrients to support all aspects of metabolism from energy production to detoxification and elimination to disease prevention. A diet rich in plenty of clean unprocessed foods with high nutrient contents is key to overall health and vitality. In short:

- ❧ Shop the perimeter of the store.
- ❧ Load up on plant-based foods (especially non-starchy vegetables).
- ❧ Make sure you are getting high-quality healthy fats and complete proteins.
- ❧ Optionally, you might want to consider adding some high-quality supplements to fill in any gaps to support healthy blood sugar, detox channels, and the metabolism.

Note: All readers are encouraged to check with your doctor before taking any herbs or supplements to determine if this is the right course for you and what would be the appropriate amount, especially those under a doctor's care or taking prescription medications.

In the next chapter, we will focus on another nutrient that is even more critical to our bodies' survival than food, and that is water.

✥ 9 ✥

Hydrate, Hydrate, Hydrate!
Dehydration May Be Slowing Your Metabolism and Making You Sick.

You are not sick, you are thirsty. Don't treat thirst with medication.
—DR. F. BATMANGHELIDJ, *Your Body's Many Cries for Water*

Composing up to 60 percent of our bodies, water is found in our blood, lymph, urine, tears, sweat, digestive tract, and brain. Each day humans lose a couple of liters of fluids from sweat, urine, breathing, and digestion. Proper hydration is fundamental to every aspect of our health and metabolism; we cannot survive longer than four days without water.

Our hydration level affects the delivery and utilization of nutrients, detoxification, and the proper functioning of every organ and tissue in the body. Water serves to lubricate and protect our joints, support digestion, regulate body temperature and pH balance, and is important for brain function and energy production.

Most people don't drink enough water each day, so they are slightly dehydrated all of the time—referred to as chronic dehydration. Drinking coffee, tea, alcohol, and sodas can actually increase your need for water because they are diuretics, which promote urine output. A CDC report indicated that 43 percent of Americans drank fewer than four cups of water daily, which is not adequate to keep up with what we excrete. Studies have shown that even slight dehydration can negatively affect our metabolic rate and lead to a myriad of symptoms including fatigue, headaches, constipation, reduced athletic performance, low energy, elevated cholesterol, dry eyes and mouth, exercise asthma, urinary tract infections, and wrinkled/sagging skin. Researchers at the University of Utah found a correlation between hydration status and metabolism.

Those in the study who drank eight glasses of water (compared to those who drank four) reported having better energy and concentration, and in general felt better. They also found that those who drank less fluids, burned fewer calories—a 3 percent dehydration status equated to a reduction in calorie burning by 2 percent.

Even mild dehydration can cause the blood to thicken, which can lead to an increased risk of a heart event. Chronic dehydration puts us at greater risk of becoming acutely dehydrated, which can be life threatening. So it is very important to our metabolism and overall health to remain properly hydrated. If you are well-hydrated, your urine should be a light lemon or straw color. Dark yellow can be an indication of dehydration (although taking a multivitamin can also discolor urine).

HORMONE HIGHLIGHTS: FLUID BALANCE

Certain hormones are involved in regulating the fluid balance in our bodies:

- **Vasopressin.** When the body is dehydrated, an anti-diuretic peptide hormone called vasopressin is released, which causes retention of water in the kidneys. It also causes constriction of the blood vessels and increases blood pressure.

- **Aldosterone.** A steroid hormone that is produced in the adrenal cortex, aldosterone helps to regulate the levels of sodium, potassium, and water in the body. It stimulates the kidneys to take in more sodium and water and to release potassium. High levels of chronic stress can stimulated and then deplete aldosterone. This is why adrenal fatigue can often lead to problems with the sodium-and-fluid balance in the body and can eventually create low blood pressure and dehydration. This is one reason people with adrenal fatigue tend to crave salt. Adding trace mineral drops of a pinch or two or high-quality unprocessed mineral-rich salts to drinking water is especially helpful for those with chronic dehydration and adrenal fatigue.

Water Quality

As with so many elements of nutrition, not all water is created equal. Water quality varies quite a bit from city to city, and therefore tap water may not be the ideal source. Just because water looks crystal clear does not mean that it is free from chemicals and toxins. There are hundreds of possible chemicals that can end up in our water supply including lead, arsenic, mercury, pesticides, industrial waste by-products, and even prescription medications. Some chemicals are purposely put into it, including fluoride and chlorine. Fluoride has been added to our drinking water for years with the goal of reducing cavities, but this practice is highly controversial and potentially linked to an increased risk of certain cancers and neurological issues. Chlorine is added to protect us from bacteria and parasites, yet there is some concern about potential health risks, including an increased cancer risk.

However, buying plastic bottled water in bulk is not the ideal solution either—from both the environmental and health perspectives. According to the Worldwatch Institute, each year over two million tons of plastic water bottles end up in landfills, and the Earth Policy Institute says that it takes about seventeen million barrels of crude oil just to produce the amount of plastic water bottles that Americans consume each year. Healthwise, the BPAs in plastic are potential hormone interrupters, so regularly drinking from plastic could lead to hormone imbalances, and as we know, healthy hormones are important for a healthy metabolism. Also, in some cases, the quality of bottled water was found to be no better than that of the tap water! In a pinch, such as when traveling, they are fine, but I do not recommend drinking water from plastic bottles for regular consumption. They are also by far the most expensive way to drink water. An economical option is to filter your water at home and drink it from a glass. There are many different systems for filtering water including reverse osmosis, activated charcoal, or carbon filters. Some can be mounted under or over the sink, while there are also whole-house and portable filtration systems and those in refrigerators.

Should We Follow Our Thirst?

Whether or not our thirst is a reliable guide for how much water we need is up for debate. Some experts believe that our bodies will tell us when we are thirsty and we should let our thirst guide us. Others claim that thirst can be a poor indicator of hydration and we need to stay ahead of our thirst and "push water." I am a big advocate of listening to our bodies, and letting them guide us—being "intuitive." But ironically, when we are chronically dehydrated, our thirst mechanism can be off. So it is a good idea to just be conscious of how much water we are drinking every day.

Shortly after rising, have an eight-ounce glass of water first thing in the morning. That alone can make a big difference! Then beyond that, a good gauge for how much water you need to drink daily is to try to consume at least half your body weight in ounces (i.e., sixty ounces daily for a 120-pound woman, or just over seven eight-ounce glasses). This is in addition to the fluids you get from the foods you eat, which should contain about two liters of fluids. Certain factors such as sweating, a hot/dry climate, a highly processed diet, and illness can increase your need for fluids. Make sure to spread your water intake out over the whole day.

Once we return our bodies to a state of optimal hydration, our thirst mechanism should be a more reliable indicator. *Note:* excessive thirst can also be a symptom of poor glucose management or diabetes. If you are extremely thirsty or have to repeatedly get up at night to go to the bathroom, you might want to have your blood glucose checked.

FASCINATING FACT

The Nobel Prize was awarded in 2003 to Peter Agre, MD, for discovering aquaporins, which are proteins within cell membranes that are responsible for the passage of water molecules across the cells. Dr. Agre called water "the solvent of life" and aquaporins, "the plumbing system for cells."

Can You Drink Too Much Water?

Yes, just like almost everything, you can get too much water. In fact, drinking a significant amount of water without replacing important electrolytes when the body is dehydrated can lead to a very dangerous condition called hyponatremia (excessively low levels of sodium in the blood). Severe cases can cause swelling in the brain, which can be deadly. Other conditions can exasperate this including Addison's disease, (advanced adrenal fatigue), diuretics, medications, heart conditions, kidney or liver disease, and more. So if there has been significant fluid loss for any reason, it is important to replenish lost electrolytes along with water.

Electrolytes are electrically charged ions that are essential for the normal functioning of our cells and organs. They are kind of like the spark plugs for our cells! If we do not have the right balance of electrolytes, we can have issues with our brain, nervous system, muscles, and more. Serious electrolyte imbalances can even lead to death. Electrolytes include sodium, potassium, chloride, bicarbonate, phosphate, magnesium, sulfate, and calcium.

Nature's Hydration Tools

Diets rich in plant-based foods provide excellent hydration because many fruits and vegetables have a high water content paired with natural electrolytes, minerals, and vitamins that are needed for hydration and cellular function. Move over sports drinks, and make room for these natural hydrators:

- **Coconut water.** Referred to as "nature's Gatorade," coconut water contains five electrolytes: sodium, potassium, magnesium, phosphorus, and calcium. It so closely matches the profile of human blood that it has been known to be used as intravenous fluid in a pinch.

- **Watermelon.** Over 90 percent water, watermelon contains calcium, magnesium, sodium, and potassium. Rich in beta-carotene, vitamin C, and lycopene, watermelon is also helpful in protecting the body from free radical damage.

- **Celery.** Crunching on celery sticks can help to return lost sodium and potassium to the body. Celery is a particularly good source of sodium. The body needs organic sodium, which works in conjunction with potassium to regulate fluids and nutrients in cells. Sodium is important for maintaining mineral balances, digestion, metabolism, nerve function, and more.

- **Cucumber.** Another high water content vegetable, cucumbers are also a good source of vitamin C and an anti-inflammatory compound called caffeic acid, which is why putting cucumber slices on your eyes can help reduce puffiness. Cucumbers are a refreshing addition to a salad and great in a fresh-pressed juice.

- ❧ **Bone broth.** A traditionally made organic bone broth with high-quality salt added is mineral rich and an excellent tool for rehydration as well as healing to the gut health.

Some other foods that, despite not being high in water content, can help to rehydrate (and even prehydrate) the body as well when paired with fluids are:

- ❧ **Chia seeds.** Chia seeds are uniquely hydrophilic, meaning each little seed can absorb approximately ten times its own weight in water. When chia seeds come into contact with fluids, they soak them up and create a gel. Chia gel can prolong hydration by retaining electrolytes and fluids in the body, making it an excellent tool for hydration. Always make sure to take chia seeds with plenty of water to ensure they are properly hydrated.

- ❧ **Sea vegetables.** Containing virtually all the minerals found in the ocean, seaweed is an excellent tool for replenishing lost minerals. Sea vegetables supply calcium, copper, iodine, iron, magnesium, manganese, molybdenum, phosphorus, potassium, selenium, vanadium, and zinc. Perhaps best known for their iodine content, sea vegetables like kelp also support the thyroid gland.

- ❧ **Fermented foods.** When foods like cucumbers and cabbage are fermented, they provide added minerals and sodium, as well as vitamins B and K, and are an excellent way to provide hydration to the body's cells.

Mineralize Your Water

One of the things I like to do is boost the mineral and electrolyte content of my daily drinking water by adding trace mineral drops to it, which can be found in most natural food markets in the supplement section. I also like to squeeze in some fresh lemon juice and add a pinch or two of unprocessed pink Himalayan salt, which helps to provide high-quality sodium, vitamin C, and trace minerals. This is especially helpful for those with adrenal fatigue, and it also supports the body to detox. However, if you have any renal disease, high blood pressure, heart disease, or diabetes, please consult your doctor first.

The Bottom Line

Chronic dehydration is very common and can be confused for hunger as well as contribute to fatigue, sluggish digestion, wrinkles, and issues with detoxification. The good news is that this is probably the easiest thing for everyone to fix: just start your day with a full glass of water and continue to drink fluids and eat more mineral-rich hydrating foods throughout your day! Your skin and cells will be more refreshed, and your metabolism will function at a higher level.

❧ 10 ❧

Exercise Smarter
(Not Harder)

Everything in physiology follows the rule that too much can be as bad as too little. . . . For example, while a moderate amount of exercise generally increases bone mass, thirty-year-old athletes who run 40 to 50 miles a week can wind up with decalcified bones, decreased bone mass, increased risk of stress fractures and scoliosis (sideways curvature of the spine)—their skeletons look like those of seventy-year-olds.

—ROBERT M. SAPOLSKY, *Why Zebras Don't Get Ulcers*

When we say that we want to lose weight, we really mean is that we want to change our body composition to be leaner (translation: we want to lose fat, not muscle). The higher percentage of muscle to fat that we have in our body, the higher our basal metabolic rate (BMR). Put simply: muscle burns more calories than fat. If you have a higher BMR, you will burn more calories, even while at rest.

Exercise is definitely an important piece of the metabolism puzzle. Regular exercise helps the body to release toxins, helps us manage stress, boosts our mood and brain functioning, and improves our insulin sensitivity (so our bodies more effectively metabolizes sugars and carbs). Exercise also creates an energy deficit and releases sugars stored in the liver and muscles (glycogen). But as with other factors in this book, not all exercise is created equal. Many people are missing the mark by either under-exercising or overexercising. Let's take a look at both ends of the exercise spectrum—and also at what really works best for our metabolism.

Sitting Is Deadly

Inactivity is terrible for the metabolism and overall health. According to the *New York Times*, a study conducted at Pennington Biomedical Research Center showed that just one day of excessive sitting can cause a 40 percent drop in the ability of insulin to uptake glucose and can slash the body's rate of calorie-burning by a third. But besides being terrible for the metabolism, sitting can be downright deadly. Studies have found that sitting for long periods increases the risk for type 2 diabetes, heart disease, and certain cancers. Research conducted by the American Cancer Society found that the death rate for men who sat more than six hours a day was 18 percent higher than for those who sat for less than three hours. For women, the risk was 37 percent! A study that looked at the National Health and Nutrition Examination Surveys found that 50 to 70 percent of people spent more than six hours each day sitting, and that eating healthy and even exercising a few times a week did not offset the damage to the body and metabolism caused by long bouts off our feet.

So what is someone to do who has to sit a lot for work? The good news is that a Mayo Clinic study discovered that even the little movements added up. Bending down to tie shoes, getting up to stretch, getting up to get some water or go to the bathroom—everything helps and adds up. So if you need to sit a lot for work or other reasons and you can't get one of those cool treadmill desks, just make sure that you get up and move around every hour. Set a timer if you need to!

Fatigue can be another reason that people sit for long periods, often relying on loved ones to "wait on them." This is a double-edged sword because the more someone sits, the more fatigued they can become. Just remember that all the little movements count. To offset this particular risk, there is no need to work out for an hour; just make sure to move a little bit every hour or so. It could be as simple as getting up to get your own glass of water, taking a short walk, or even helping with the dishes after dinner.

Too Much of a Good Thing?

There are also lots of people who are not couch potatoes at all. In fact, they are working really hard to stay in shape. They are regulars at the gym, part of a running group, or hit the treadmill four to five days a week. Yet despite working out regularly, the weight around their midsection just won't budge! If you are in this category, I have good news for you—you could be working out *too hard.*

We often think that if a little is good, then more is better. But this is not necessarily true, especially when it comes to cardiovascular exercise. Our bodies are not designed to run marathons. We evolved from hunter-gatherers, who very rarely just sat around, but they also didn't run twenty-six miles at once. They ran as far and as fast as they needed to get out of harm's way. Hunter-gatherers had short bursts of intense cardio, mixed in with some heavy lifting, and lots of little movements in between. From an evolutionary standpoint, our bodies, long bouts of cardio are a source of chronic *stress.* As we know, stress raises our stress hormones—including cortisol levels—which tell our bodies to store fat, especially in our midsection. They also steal from our other hormones, increase inflammation, and disrupt our digestion. Bingo! That could explain why working out harder and running longer could add up to weight gain and other issues. It is the cortisol hard at work , storing fat right in our midsection. What's the other thing that too much cardio can do? Break down muscle and bone, and accelerate aging.

The metabolism has two opposing phases: Anabolism is building, and catabolism is breaking down. We need both for homeostasis. But if we are overtraining, especially doing too much cardio, there can be too much catabolism, which can lead to a loss of muscle and bone mass. This is not good for the metabolism. Excess catabolism can also increase the physical signs of aging—not the typical goals we have when we sign up for a gym membership!

Smarter Exercise

Working out smarter, not necessarily longer and harder, is the key to a healthy metabolism and getting rid of that pesky midsection bulge. Our exercise needs to do two things:

1. Keep our stress hormones from firing off all the time (don't overdo the cardio, include some rest and recovery, yoga or meditation).

2. Build or protect lean muscle tissue (include some weight-bearing exercises).

One of the most effective ways to exercise for a healthy metabolism is to do short bursts of cardio, followed by low-intensity cardio and/or weight training, commonly referred to as interval training or high-intensity interval training (HIIT). HIIT is composed of as little as thirty seconds of very intense cardio interspersed with two to four minutes of low-intensity or weight-bearing exercises and repeating this cycle about four to five times. A study conducted at Heriot-Watt University in Edinburgh found that after just two weeks of exercising this way, participants were able to improve insulin sensitivity, which means the cells are responding appropriately to insulin. The cool thing about HIIT is that it is an effective solution for people who only have ten to fifteen minutes to exercise.

I recommend a full checkup before you embark on a fitness program, especially with a high level of intensity. HIIT may not be safe for those with an existing medical condition.

Why Yoga Is Good for Our Metabolism

Studies show that people who practice yoga tend to be a healthier weight than those who do not. One of the likely reasons could be because it lowers our stress hormone cortisol. Another could be because it fosters mindfulness. When we are mindful, we tend to make healthier choices. Mindfulness helps us to connect to how our bodies feel and function after certain foods, so we will make better choices.

Extreme Dieting Backfires

When we drastically cut calories and drop weight really fast, there can be muscle loss along with fat loss. Because drastic calorie restriction slows down the metabolism, when we go off the diet, the weight can easily be gained back (85 percent of dieters gain the weight back). If there has been muscle loss, we end up gaining that lost muscle back as fat. This is how yo-yo dieting can make us fatter and sicker in the long run.

The Bottom Line

Over- or under-exercising are both detrimental to the metabolism. One critical thing to avoid is sitting for long periods of time, which causes our metabolism to crash and burn. But the other side of the spectrum can backfire too: Excess cardio can raise cortisol levels, which prompts our bodies to store fat in our midsection and break down muscle. Finding the right type and level of exercise for you is a key piece of the metabolism puzzle.

✥ 11 ✥

Metabolism Hacks
Timing Might Be Everything

If five to six meals a day are needed to maintain energy, the metabolic situation is not in good shape.

—BYRON RICHARDS, CCN, author of *Mastering Leptin: Your Guide to Permanent Weight Loss and Health*

Google the word "metabolism" and many of the articles that pop up will say that you need to "eat every couple of hours" to keep your metabolism "up." But that advice can easily backfire because too often, we are eating simple carbs and sugars every couple of hours. As we know, a typical snack of carbohydrates causes insulin to be released, which tells our body to store those excess calories as fat. Doing that every couple of hours all day long, never gives our body the chance to go into fat-burning mode because it is stuck in sugar-burning/fat-storage mode. You can see how frequent snacking can be a recipe for metabolism meltdown. According to a paper published in the *British Journal of Nutrition*, "A detailed review of the possible mechanistic explanations for a metabolic advantage of nibbling meal patterns failed to reveal significant benefits in respect of energy expenditure."

Sticking to three square meals a day may in fact be better because it allows for the body to enter into fat-burning mode in between meals. The body can't transition to fat-burning mode if it is stuck in sugar-burning mode, which can happen when someone is snacking all day long. Some people might even want to consider exploring how to take timing to the next level—to in a sense "hack" their metabolism.

What Is Intermittent Fasting?

A new trend in the nutrition world is based on the centuries-old tradition of fasting. Intermittent fasting (IF) devotees say that not only does IF boost energy and metabolism, but it also reduces disease risk factors. IF basically means having a period of time when you do not eat followed by a period of time when you do. In fact, we are all engaged in IF every time we go to bed, because unless we are eating in our sleep, we are fasting for as long as we are snoozing. That is why our first meal of the day is called breakfast, because it "breaks the fast."

But the big benefits of intermittent fasting start to kick in when you extend that normal fasting window, say from eight or ten hours, to fourteen to sixteen hours. This gives us an eight- to ten-hour window in which to eat, as popularized in *The Eight Hour Diet*, by David Zinczenko and Peter Moore. That could look like eating your first meal at 9 a.m. and your last at 5 or 7 p.m. Some people might choose instead to fast for twenty-four hours once a week or once a month, and then eat regularly on the other days. Another popular method of IF is to have two very low-calorie days (only about 500 calories for women or 600 calories for men) and then eat normally for the other five, sometimes referred to as the 5:2 diet. This is the type of IF promoted by Dr. Michael Mosely in *The Fast Diet*.

Scientists at the Salk Institute in La Jolla found that mice who ate within an eight-hour window were healthier than another group of mice fed the same diet who could eat at their leisure throughout the day. The study found that after 100 days, the mice who ate at will gained weight and had high cholesterol, elevated blood glucose, liver damage, and diminished motor control, but the mice in the time-restricted feeding group had no health issues, weighed 28 percent less, and performed better on an exercise test. According to the study, the mechanism for how restricted feeding works is that the body stores fat when eating and only goes into fat-burning mode a few hours after eating, at which time cholesterol is also metabolized. Study authors said that because the study was done on mice, the results may not transfer to humans, and they also cautioned against using IF alone to manage weight. A healthy diet should accompany it. Regardless, it sheds some light on the possibility that frequent eating could be a major player in the battle of the bulge, and that IF, when combined with other key factors, could be another powerful way to support a healthy metabolism.

Is IF for Everyone?

You might want to think seriously before jumping on the IF bandwagon, however. IF may not be appropriate for everyone (such as endurance athletes, people with blood sugar control issues, diabetes, heart disease, adrenal fatigue, or another health condition),because it could lead to dangerously low drops in blood sugar. Other studies have also come to different conclusions than the Salk Institute study. One Harvard study found that men who skipped breakfast were 27 percent more likely to experience a heart attack. One reason that skipping breakfast might be bad is that it could put the body in a state of stress, which could disrupt the metabolism and amplify other health risk factors. But it was not entirely clear if skipping breakfast *caused* the increase or was just *correlated*. More research needs to be done in this area. Just realize that IF may not be appropriate for everyone, or might not be suited for a long duration.

I think the key point to take away from this is that it is important to listen to your body. If you do better with a snack or two, look for options that will keep the blood sugar from spiking and dropping. Make sure to use the Rule of Three to balance out your blood sugar with healthy fat, fiber, and/or protein. One of my favorite snacks? A half (or whole) avocado with some lime juice and salt sprinkled on it. Sometimes I will mash it up and spread it on cucumber slices. Another really easy snack is a water bottle filled with filtered water, chia seeds, protein powder, and a greens packet—I call it a *Quick Pick-Me-Up Drink!*

And don't feel like you need to go to the extreme either. It turns out that just keeping your window of eating to twelve hours and sticking with three square meals a day may offer good metabolism benefits, because your body gets several shorts fasts during the day to burn fat and a longer one at night. The most important thing is to listen to your body and make good decisions about when and what to eat, which can change based on your activity, sleep, stress levels, and other factors.

Do Carbs Have a Time and a Place?

As you know by now, snacking on sugar and simple carbs all day long spikes insulin over and over, which tells the body to store fat rather than lose it. Over time, a chronically elevated blood sugar level can lead to insulin resistance, stubborn weight gain, and a higher risk of many diseases. So sugars and starchy carbs are bad for the metabolism, and we should keep them as low as possible, right?

Well, as with many other keys in this book, it is not that simple. . . .

There is a yin and yang to carbohydrates. On the one side, yes, eating too many simple carbs can get the metabolism "stuck" in sugar-burning, fat storage mode. This is not good for the metabolism or disease risk. However, cutting carbs too low or for too long can end up backfiring too. For certain individuals, diets that are extremely low in carbohydrates over time can make the thyroid sluggish, increase stress hormones, interfere with sleep, break down muscle tissue, and squash sex hormone and neurotransmitter levels. That's not exactly the picture of health either.

Now wait just one minute! We need to cut back on carbs to get out of fat-storage mode, but if we do it too drastically or for too long, our hormones and our metabolism might suffer? Yep. So what exactly should we do then?

That's another million dollar question! The answer has two parts:

The first step to fixing the metabolism is to get the body out of sugar-burning mode. This is done by decreasing sugars and high glycemic foods, increasing your healthy fats, eating more vegetables, and getting plenty of high-quality proteins. You will know if you are out of sugar-burning mode if you have begun to release excess weight, you are able to go for four hours in between meals and not get "hangry" (hungry angry), and you are feeling energized, less moody, and are sleeping better.

The second step, once the body is in fat-burning mode, is to find the optimal balance of carbs *for you*, to ensure that you are properly feeding hormones, energy, neurotransmitters, muscles, brain, etc., yet not enough to put you right back into sugar-burning mode (this happens in phase four of the Perfect Metabolism plan—your forever phase). If you find your energy, mood, brain function, and sleep are starting to suffer, you probably need to add another serving of carbs. Did you work out particularly hard? Are you under a lot of stress? All of these things can change your body's requirements for carbs, other macronutrients, and micronutrients.

Carbohydrate consumption is another area where it appears that timing might matter. Eating the lion's share of our carbohydrates in the morning seems like it would be better for our metabolism, because carbs supply energy during the day when we need it and we can also "burn them off by exercising." Having carbs at night sounds bad because we can't burn them off while we sleep, so logic tells us that will just go "straight to our waistline." But a 2012 study at the Hebrew University of Jerusalem found exactly the opposite to be true. A group of police officers with a body mass index (BMI) over thirty were put on identical low calorie diets. One group spread their carbohydrate intake throughout the day, while the other group ate them all at dinner. The group that ate their carbs at dinner lost more weight, reported less hunger, and showed improved blood sugar and other metabolic effects.

It turns out that there are several benefits that carbs supply, some of which are boosted by eating most of them at dinner:

- Carbohydrates support sleep. An Australian study showed that consuming higher glycemic carbohydrates four hours before bedtime helped study participants fall asleep faster. *As we know, a good night's sleep is very important for balancing hormones, stress levels, cellular repair and detoxification, and overall metabolism.*

- They support the adrenal glands and neurotransmitters, which are important brain chemicals. So anyone with adrenal fatigue is going to want to make sure that they are not cutting their carbs too low.

- With the right kinds and in the right amounts, in people with a healthy digestive system, carbohydrates can support a healthy gut bacterial balance. Carbohydrates supply fiber, which is important for digestion and to serve as food for our good bacteria.

- According to the Jerusalem study, eating carbohydrates at dinnertime improved leptin, ghrelin, and adiponectin levels—three very important hormones that drive appetite, fat-burning, and satiation. Study participants who ate the majority of carbs at night also improved their blood sugar levels and markers for inflammation, and shrunk their waist more.

So if you want to maximize your carbohydrates, save the starchy carbs and higher glycemic foods for your evening meal. Ideally focus primarily on getting plenty of healthy fat (nuts, seeds, avocado, coconut), high-quality proteins (chicken, beef, pork, nuts, eggs if using), and as many non-starchy vegetables as you like during the day. Need a small serving of berries or some quinoa on your salad? Go for it, but limit them to a small serving and eat them with protein or fat to lower the glycemic response. Dinnertime is ideal for adding in a serving of one of the following: sweet potato, yam, pumpkin, squash (winter, acorn, and butternut), artichokes, plantains, beets, legumes, green beans, carrots, buckwheat, quinoa, basmati or jasmine rice, rice pasta, amaranth, or tapioca, or a food made with a nongluten flour. You might even find that, despite being a very high glycemic food, a white potato once in a while works for you. You might even enjoy a glass of wine with dinner a few nights a week. Consider reading the book *The Carb Nite Solution* by John Keifer if you are interested in exploring this approach to eating further.

The Bottom Line

People ask me all the time what I think of this or that new supplement that is supposedly the latest and greatest "miracle" weight loss tool. My response is that although there certainly are some supplements that can support or even jump-start their metabolism, they should be skeptical if someone promises a "magic pill" that will replace a healthy diet and balanced exercise regimen. In fact, because metabolism is all about balance, it is possible to overstimulate it with supplements. However, there is good evidence to support that short periods of fasting and the proper amount and timing of carbohydrates can "hack" our metabolism naturally.

Just remember that everyone is unique and different. When it comes to the timing of your meals, whether you need a snack, or the amount and timing of your carbs, there is no one-size-fits-all approach. The right timing and amount will be based on individual needs, which can change from day to day. For example, on days that you exercise, you will need slightly more carbs than when you do not. Once we move through the three phases in the next part of the book and reach your forever phase, you will be doing some "investigative work" of your own about what is best for you. You will want to check in regularly with yourself to assess your energy, mood, hunger, and brain function. Make sure to listen to your body. It is all about finding the right balance for *your* healthy metabolism.

Part Two

Take Action! The Perfect Metabolism Cleanse

Create Your Perfect Metabolism!

Now it is time to put the keys from part one into action to unlock and create your Perfect Metabolism! This section guides you on how to implement the keys to reboot your metabolism and regain your vitality.

Perfect Metabolism is not a calorie-restrictive juice fast or a master cleanse. It is a nourishing, gentle, and fulfilling foods-based program designed to help reboot your metabolism. It does involve some cooking, but don't worry if you are not big on working in the kitchen. Many people who have done this program have totally surprised themselves (and their families) with their cooking skills! I can tell you from my own personal experience, the more you cook, the easier and more enjoyable it becomes.

Planning ahead is one key to success. Sit down every couple of days, select the recipes you want to make, get to the store, and do the necessary prep ahead of time.

Over the next three-plus weeks, you will be gradually making changes in your life and implementing the Perfect Metabolism keys. But remember, each of us is unique. For some people, this will be a huge departure and complete overhaul. For others, it will be more of a minor tune-up. Just be gentle with yourself. If you need longer to move forward, then please take your time.

The Perfect Metabolism Cleanse is done in three phases:

Phase One: **ReSet** is designed to help you mentally and physically prepare. We'll start with some simple changes, like getting the sugar out, fixing your fats, and easing off of certain foods. Listen to your heart and your body, be mindful and gentle, and make good choices for yourself. Take one week or longer if you need to.

Phase Two is the **ReBoot** and will last approximately one to two weeks (or longer if you wish). In this phase you'll be eating highly nourishing and cleansing foods, avoiding toxins, supporting digestion and elimination, etc. You should not feel deprived during this phase; rather your body should experience being deeply nourished and cared for. Once you stop introducing new toxins, your body will start to clean house and get rid of old waste products. You will be supporting this process by eating lots of fibrous, seasonal vegetables and fruits and increasing your fluid intake.

The third phase is **ReIntroduce,** which should last another one to two weeks. During this phase, you will systematically try out the foods that were eliminated in phases one and two to identify sensitivities. Ideally, you should wait at least twenty-four hours before reintroducing the next food, which is why this phase can sometimes take a little longer.

In phase four, you will **ReNew—Merge/Move On.** This is the forever phase. You should feel revitalized, rejuvenated, clearer-headed, and full of new knowledge about yourself. Hopefully you won't jump back into old patterns but instead be excited about a "new" normal, where you will continue to incorporate more plant-based foods, organics, and healthy fats. You will continue to avoid the foods that were not serving you, such as foods that you are intolerant to and processed convenience foods.

❧ 12 ❧

Phase One
ReSet

This first phase is designed to allow you to ease into the program, mentally and physically. You will do some planning and prep work, begin to ease off certain foods, and start to implement some of the Perfect Metabolism keys. Change is not easy, especially habits that have formed over many years or many decades, so use this week to allow the body and mind to adjust.

As you increase the healthy fats, get rid of the sugar, and ease off the toxic junk foods, your cravings will begin to diminish.

Consider the following as you embark on a new set of habits:

- ❧ If you are not used to eating a lot of fiber, gradually increase your intake by adding one to two servings of plant-based foods daily. You might want to begin with lightly steamed veggies, which can be easier to digest. Start with one to two teaspoons of well-hydrated chia seeds, and if that is okay, gradually work your way up to two tablespoons.

- ❧ Increase your water/fluid intake to support digestion, elimination, and detoxification. Start each morning with a full glass of water, and shoot for half your body weight in ounces for your daily fluid intake.

- ❧ If you drink a lot of coffee, this is the week to start cutting back or replacing some with green tea. You can go to half decaf (*just make sure that you are using Swiss Water Process decaf coffee*).

- ❧ If you rely on wine to settle you down at night, this is the week to begin to rein that back. If that freaks you out, consider taking 500 mg. of glutamine and.or 100 mg. of L-theanine in the late afternoon.

- Are you a soda drinker, or do you crave chips and fast foods? Remember that these foods rob your body of nutrients, burden the liver, and steal your energy. Try to ease off of them and replace them with high-quality healthy fats, proteins, and fiber-rich plant foods.

- Look at your commitments over the next three weeks. Are there some things that can be pushed off until later? Reducing your obligations can help you stay focused on your health goals.

In the first phase you may begin to incorporate some of the Perfect Metabolism recipes (see chapter sixteen) and principles each day while you work on weaning yourself off the elimination foods and drinks. Try to find time each day to relax and get some "soul food". Allow time each day for some planning and prep: that is the key to success in the kitchen. Some goals for this week:

- Set up your environment for success (get rid of temptations).

- Start to build awareness (read labels, journal to track feelings, etc.).

- Get the sugar and junk out. (I promise you will feel so much better soon!)

- Fix your fats (they fill you up and keep you satisfied).

- Begin to ease off/eliminate some key foods and drinks.

- Gradually increase the fiber and plant-based foods in your daily diet.

- Become aware of and begin to reduce exposure to toxins and chemicals.

Action Items

Clean Out the Pantry/Build Awareness

If we are surrounded by temptations, it is hard to stick to a plan. So it is time to clean the pantry and get those trigger foods out of the house. This also makes it clear how much sugar, high glycemic carbs, trans fats, and processed ingredients we are really eating. If you have not been much of a label reader, now is the time to put on your nutrition detective cap and start to study those labels. This can be eye-opening and a critical step in long-term health!

Keep your eye on the prize: once we get all the metabolic dominoes lined up and working optimally and the hunger hormones come into balance, it becomes *less of an effort* to make good choices:

- We have fewer cravings.
- We are more satisfied after we eat.
- Super sweet things don't taste as good as they used to.
- We have longer-lasting energy and are less likely to need to "grab anything."

But until that kicks in, we need to hit the override button and rely on some of that good old-fashioned willpower while identifying and removing our trigger foods.

"Trigger foods" are like kryptonite: they spike hunger and cravings. Get them out of your house, so you will not be tempted. Be honest with yourself about what your trigger foods are. One of mine is still pretzels (yes, even gluten-free ones!). Sometimes there is an "upgrade" option, so you can swap a troublesome food for something better. For example, Mary's Gone Crackers are an *upgraded* pretzel: they are gluten-free and contain chia seeds and whole grains, so I will be less likely to overeat them.

Here are some investigative tips:

- **Read the label.** Does it have sugar in there? How many different types/names? Is it the first, second, or third ingredient? Scrutinize anything with more than one type of sugar or more than six grams of sugar (that is 1.5 teaspoons).

  If high fructose corn syrup (HFCS) is on the label, I always look for another option. HFCS is highly processed and typically made from genetically modified corn. It is a cheap ingredient, so the other ingredients are also probably cheap and/or GMO too.

- **Are you buying cereals, sports bars, and muffins?** Those can be sneaky sources of sugar (as well as GMO corn and soy). I have lots of busy clients who come to me with digestive issues and weight gain, and many of them don't realize that it could be the bars they have been eating. If you need a bar, look for one with no soy, gluten, or dairy and less than eight grams of sugar. (Yes, that is two teaspoons. Remember, the AHA wants women not to exceed six teaspoons and men should be at or under nine teaspoons.)

- **Check your fridge.** Other sneaky places sugar is hiding are in those bottles of condiments, sauces, marinades, and dressings. When you go to the store, compare labels. Does the barbecue sauce you usually get have tomatoes as the first ingredient? Or is it high fructose corn syrup? Believe it or not, there are *lots* of brands that have more sugar than tomatoes in them! The same goes with salad dressings; many have sugar as the first or second ingredient, and most contain unhealthy forms of fat too.

- **Are you adding sugar to your foods (like coffee, tea, oatmeal)?** Try to wean off the sweets by using a little bit of stevia or coconut sugar. Eventually try to go without them altogether.

Get Them Out! Eliminate Metabolism-Busting Foods

Time to pitch or pack up and put away sweets, high glycemic foods, and processed foods. They spike your hunger, slow down your metabolism, and tell your body to store fat—right in your midsection.

The things to get rid of are:

- Sugary snacks—cereal bars, cookies, granola bars, etc.

- Sweetened drinks—sodas, sweet lattes, sweet teas, sports drinks, energy drinks

- Gum—yes both sugar-free and regular—because it all can contain artificial sweeteners, colors, and flavors or petroleum. Some people can also be bothered by xylitol.

- Wine, beer, other alcoholic beverages (yep, sorry, it's timeto give the liver a break!)

- Breads (except "Paleo" or perhaps an occasional slice of gluten-free bread)

- Pretzels and most snacky foods

- White potatoes, chips

- Ice cream, popsicles, frozen desserts

- Frozen waffles, pancakes, pizzas

- Candy (except the chocolate recipes in this book or dark chocolate that has a cacao content of 70 percent or more)
- Cakes, baked goods, muffins
- Dairy products (all cow's milk products)
- Highly processed, enriched foods (most packaged foods)
- Foods with artificial colors, flavors, MSG, dough conditioners, or other chemicals
- Anything that says low fat, reduced fat, sugar free, or "diet"
- Unhealthy fats including corn oil, canola oil, soy oil, cottonseed oil, vegetable oil, margarines, or anything with trans fats (partially hydrogenated oils)
- Bottled dressings (especially those with sugar, MSG, or unhealthy fats)
- White table salt

Replacements for the Above Foods

- Kombucha (a fermented tea beverage which is a good alternative to sodas)
- Milk alternatives: almond, coconut, cashew, hemp, flax (unsweetened)
- Pink Himalayan, Celtic, or naturally air-dried sea salt
- Gluten-free alternatives to grains like quinoa, buckwheat, teff, amaranth, and millet
- Flour alternatives: nut (almond, cashew), coconut, and garbanzo bean
- Homemade salad dressings (see the recipes in chapter sixteen)
- Lots of fresh vegetables

Wait! What if you need to keep some of these things in the house for other family members? You could ask them to help you out by stashing them somewhere where you won't be tempted by them . . . or maybe they are game to clean up their diets right alongside you!

Get Shopping!

Now that you have gotten the temptations and toxic foods out of the cabinet and refrigerator, it is time to shop! Look through the recipes in chapter sixteen, and decide which ones you want to try. Write up your shopping list, and get to the store. I recommend that you stock up on pantry staples and buy the fresh ingredients needed for the next three days. Now remember, this is our ease-in phase, so don't feel like you have to do it all at once. You can ramp this up gradually over this week or longer. You can also substitute other recipes; just stick to the guidelines.

Find shopping lists and meal plans at *www.perfectmetabolism.com*.

Write Your Breakup Letter

Are you ready to get sugar out of your life? Or is there something holding you back?

Even if we know that a relationship is not good for us and is wreaking havoc on our life, it is still not easy to say good-bye. Maybe there is a part of you that just doesn't want to give it up. That is totally normal. Like most people, your relationship with sugar probably goes way back. Most relationships start out good—amazing, actually. They bring something positive to our lives. They make us happy. But if a relationship starts to become unhealthy, we need to take inventory. So let's get a closer look at the one we have with sugar (in all forms).

Here is my breakup letter:

Dear Sugar,

I used to love you very deeply. I don't think I even realized how much I loved you! You were always there for me anytime I needed a pick-me-up. You brought a wonderful sweetness into my life. I have many happy memories of our time together—baking cookies with my sister (which truthfully was more about eating the dough than baking it), frozen yogurt with candy swirled in, Baskin-Robbins peanut butter and chocolate on a sugar cone, the fizzy sodas at the movies, the pillowcase full of Halloween candy, and Grammy's Christmas fudge. I could go on and on. You made me happy—giddy, really.

But alas, you came with a price—weight gain, moodiness, diges-tion issues, cravings, serious fatigue, brain fog, immune issues, and much more. Being with you was like being on a roller coaster! The time has come. I think the nail in the coffin was when I found out that you were making me look older (boy, do I wish I knew about that one a little earlier)! I have come to realize that I can no longer pay the price—you are just not worth it.

Don't try to talk me out of it. I have moved on. Recently, I have been spending a lot of time with someone else. I am just going to come right out and say it—it is FAT. I used to run away from fat. I had been told for so long that fat was part of the "bad crowd." But now I realize that I was so very wrong. I am not alone; more people are starting to realize that fat's poor reputation is undeserved. Like most relationships, it's not all roses. Fat does have some family members that I avoid like the plague (the dangerous trans fats, and that motley crew of soy, corn, and canola oils—they are just too unstable and mostly genetically modified). But for the most part, my relationship with fat is everything I have been looking for and more. . . . I know I shouldn't play favorites, but I can't help it—coconut is by far my favorite.

I want you to know that I couldn't be happier now. Fat has made my life so wonderful. Instead of sweetness, I am enjoying rich creaminess. Fat is my rock—instead of a roller coaster. I am stable—my feet are firmly planted on the solid ground. Instead of cravings, I am satisfied. Instead of moodiness, I feel calm and centered. I have even noticed a difference when I look in the mirror. My reflection is decidedly less wrinkled and tired. My skin looks more plump and rested. And I am happy to say that I have found a way to have my cake and eat it too. I met some of your cousins— stevia, coconut sugar, raw honey, and lo han guo. They are pretty cool because when I want just a little sweetness in my life, they are there for me and don't leave me feeling empty, sad, and tired. And I don't get all out of control with them like I did with you, sugar.

Listen, it's not you, it's me. I've changed. Since we have been apart for a while, I have found that less is more. . . . I have become more sensitive. Those ice creams, cookie dough, and fudge I used to dream about are just too sweet—they aren't even appealing to me anymore!

Let's face it, sugar, we've had some good times, but the peaks were followed by valleys that kept getting deeper. The bad times just finally got to me. I knew it was time to move on. There are millions of people who still love you, sugar, so I know you won't be lonely. I know there will be times that I might be tempted by you in the future. But as long as fat is in the picture, my new love keeps me feeling satisfied, strong, and stable. Once in a blue moon, we'll see each other, because the occasional small bowl of gelato might be in my cards . . . but only the really good (full-fat) kind and never again doused in caramel or topped with candy!

So good-bye for now. I don't regret our time or hold a grudge (well, except maybe a little one for those darn wrinkles). There will always be a place in my history for you, but it is just that—history.

STAY SWEET,
SARA

I encourage you to write your break up letter to sugar. Post it somewhere you can look at it every day, or when you are reaching for your sugar "fix."

Fix Your Fats

Make sure that you are increasing the amount of healthy fats you are getting (while decreasing the simple carbs and sugar). Healthy fats are critical to get rid of sugar cravings and turn off our hunger signals. *Just remember that even healthy fats can get stored as fat if you are eating them with high glycemic carbs.*

1. **Virgin coconut oil.** My absolute favorite healthy fat is unrefined virgin coconut oil. I view coconut oil not only as a healthy oil for cooking and recipes, but I also use it like a supplement. I find that if I do not have coconut oil in the morning, I crave more carbs all day long.

   ◆ How to take coconut oil? I like to add a teaspoon or two to my tea, smoothie, or coffee (if I am not in phase two) in the morning. Use coconut oil for cooking. I love to sauté veggies in it. Also check out the recipe section for some yummy coconut oil recipes. Start with one teaspoon of coconut oil in the morning and evening. Work up to two teaspoons morning and evening (you can also take an extra teaspoon or two in a cup of herbal tea if you crave sugar).

2. **Chia seeds.** Quite possibly the perfect superfood, chia seeds boost endurance, energy, hydration, focus/attention, and reduce hunger and inflammation. Chia seeds are a rich source of the ALA form of omega-3 fatty acids, which is why I have them listed under fats. But they also contain a very unique hydrophilic fiber—which basically means they soak up a lot of liquid—like ten times their own weight! This creates a chia gel, which fills us up, keeps us hydrated, and slows the absorption of sugar into the bloodstream! Always make sure to consume chia seeds with plenty of water or liquids to prevent dehydration.

   ◆ Add chia seeds to your smoothie, make chia pudding, or just add them to fresh-pressed juice, water, or a dairy alternative for a snack or energy boost. Hydrated chia seeds also support healthy digestion.

3. **Avocados.** These are full of healthy fats that help to reduce inflammation, boost the absorption of fat-soluble vitamins, and are also a high-fiber food! Avocados are a good source of carotenoids, vitamin K, vitamins B5 and B6, vitamin C, folate, and potassium. Avocados have been shown to help manage blood sugar. One half to one whole avocado a day is a great way to increase your healthy fats and fiber in your diet!

   ◆ I sometimes will just eat an avocado with a spoon for a snack after squeezing a little lime or lemon in it and sprinkling with Himalayan salt! That definitely lasts me longer than a handful of pretzels. Try adding avocados to your salad, alongside eggs, or to your smoothie. Avocados make smoothies light and fluffy, boost the fiber and vitamin content, and help to keep you satisfied longer. Avocado oil is a very versatile oil too. It has a high smoking point, so it is an ideal cooking oil. The mild taste is great in salad dressings, pestos, and more.

4. **Organic grass-fed ghee**. A type of clarified butter that has been used in Indian and Ayurvedic cooking for centuries, ghee is considered a healing and sacred food. It is very stable and has

a high smoke point (about 485 degrees), so it will not oxidize easily. It is technically "dairy based," but the milk solids have been removed during the clarification. Because most casein and lactose have been removed, ghee is less likely than other dairy products to cause digestive issues. But because there may be trace amounts of casein and lactose, very sensitive individuals will want to avoid it and choose another option. Ghee does not require refrigeration unless you do not plan to use it all within three months, then it is best to store in the refrigerator.

Pitch the Unhealthy Fats

The fats that can't be fixed are:

- **Pro-inflammatory fats** such as vegetable, canola, cottonseed, corn, and soy oils, margarine.

- **Soy oil.** Even if you are not buying soy oil, if you are eating packaged and processed foods, mayonnaise, or salad dressings, then you are probably getting soy oil.

- **Corn oil.** It is often eye-opening to find out how much corn is really in our diets. It is in so many packaged and processed foods. And high fructose corn syrup? Yep, made with corn.

- **Hydrogenated and partially hydrogenated oils.** All man-made trans fats *must* be avoided.

- **Margarine.** This butter substitute is full of trans fats. Just use the real stuff—grass-fed butter or, better yet, ghee.

Ease into the Food Elimination

During this first phase, you will begin to *gradually* ease off some foods/substances. *Take as long as you need to do this.* You will know you are ready to move on to phase two when you are ready to go at least seven days without the elimination foods. We need to remove them at least that long in order to "challenge" them back in and notice if there is a reaction/possible intolerance.

Foods to eliminate:

1. Sugar/artificial sweeteners
2. Wheat/gluten

3. Dairy (*keep in grass-fed ghee if you like*)

4. Soy

5. Corn

6. Alcohol

7. Coffee

8. *Eggs* (optional)

Going Wheat- and Gluten-Free

With so many people now limiting gluten, the gluten-free options available to you have never been better. But remember, just because a product is gluten-free does not mean it is healthy. In fact, many gluten-free products are high in sugar and contain GMO ingredients or a lot of starches, and they can be low in fiber and protein. When going gluten-free, look for products with simple ingredients, whole grains, and superfoods like flax and chia seeds.

Some healthier gluten-free swaps:

- Quinoa
- Alternative flours (almond, coconut, brown rice, buckwheat, millet, quinoa, garbanzo bean, and teff)
- Legumes (ideally sprouted or soaked lentils, black beans, white beans, garbanzo beans)
- Spaghetti squash or zucchini "noodles" are both great alternatives to pasta
- Sweet potatoes, yams, squash
- Nongluten grains in moderation: brown rice, white rice, jasmine rice, black rice, certified gluten-free oats, whole grain teff, gluten-free bread Limit yourself to one serving of any of the aforementioned per day ideally. If active, add one more starchy vegetable or grain serving. Keep in mind:
    - Almost all protein/meats are gluten-free (except those cold meats and processed meats that have gluten added).
    - Lettuce wraps are a great option in place of buns, bread, and tortillas or wraps—*butter lettuce and chard work great.*
- Eat salads instead of sandwiches.

Foods to avoid:

- ❧ Wheat
- ❧ Barley
- ❧ Rye
- ❧ Non-certified gluten-free oats
- ❧ Bulgur
- ❧ Couscous
- ❧ Orzo
- ❧ Panko
- ❧ Spelt
- ❧ Udon
- ❧ Beer
- ❧ Soy sauce
- ❧ Monosodium glutamate (MSG) and hydrolyzed vegetable proteins
- ❧ Deli meats and processed meats with gluten, nitrates, or other preservatives (read the label)
- ❧ Flours made from wheat or gluten grains (and foods made with them like gravies or soups)
- ❧ Anything breaded
- ❧ Many processed foods can have added gluten.
- ❧ Some other unexpected sources of wheat and gluten: medications, supplements, personal care products. Always check your labels.

Going Dairy-Free

I do purchase and use nondairy milks from the store, but I prefer to make my own whenever possible. Not only do they taste absolutely delicious and are quite easy to make, some of the ones you buy at the store contain additives that bother some people's digestive system, like carrageenan. In chapter sixteen, you will find several recipes for coconut, cashew, and almond milk (I even offer an easy and super quick "cheaters" version).

Dairy foods to avoid:

- ✿ Cow's milk as well as goat and sheep milk (Some people might choose to keep goat or sheep milk in because it tends to be easier on the digestion/metabolism. However, others will want to eliminate all forms of dairy.)

- ✿ Cheese, including cream and cottage

- ✿ Yogurt

- ✿ Cream

- ✿ Whey protein

Some nondairy milk alternatives are:

- ✿ Coconut

- ✿ Almond

- ✿ Cashew

- ✿ Flax

- ✿ Hemp

I do not recommend soy milk at all, because it has high levels of phytic acids, is difficult to digest, and contains phytoestrogens.

Cutting Out the Coffee? It's All about the Adrenals and Acidity

Coffee is one of those foods that people have a passion about. So many of us love our coffee! I know, I am right there with you. It is more than just a drink, it is like a good friend—comforting and energizing at the same time. In many ways coffee is very good for us. It contains antioxidants, and multiple studies show that it is linked with a reduction in the risk for many diseases including diabetes, depression, Parkinson's, and dementia or Alzheimer's. It can boost our metabolic rate and could also support the liver. So with all those positive things about coffee, why should we give it up?

There are some downsides to coffee. First, the caffeine can be overstimulating to the adrenals and can raise our cortisol levels. Coffee is acidifying and dehydrating. Taking a short break from coffee is an excellent way to improve hydration, support the adrenals, improve sleep, and balance the body's pH. Just know that this does not mean that you must give up coffee forever—it is about taking a *short break*.

Do I have you convinced? The decision is up to you.

I never thought I could give it up. But swapping it for green tea when I led my very first Perfect Metabolism program was enlightening. I was sleeping better, I felt less dehydrated and acidic, and my overall energy level was better. But despite all that, when I am on my "forever plan," I still do like to have a cup of joe; I just try to not rely on it every day. I enjoy it a few times a week with some coconut cream and a teaspoon of coconut oil in it. Other days, I will have a cup of green tea.

A wonderful alternative to coffee, green tea offers loads of antioxidants and contains L-theanine, which boosts focus and lowers anxiety. I also like pu-erh tea. It has a dark rich color, so it is very similar to coffee. And it is known to support digestion and boost the metabolism, which is one reason pu-erh is sometimes called "diet tea." I recommend organic loose-leaf teas over tea bags. The bonus with loose tea is that you can re-steep the same leaves several times. Oolong tea is another nice option. I recommend limiting intake to a few cups a day, as teas can also be dehydrating if overconsumed.

Herbal coffee substitutes—such as Dandy Blend and Teeccino—are nice options too (make sure you are choosing a gluten-free variety). They taste a lot like coffee but have no caffeine and are not acidifying. Cacao tea is a wonderful option too, since it has the dark richness of coffee and a hint of chocolate! Find what works for you, and make the change gradually, so your body has time to adjust and you don't end up with a splitting headache.

Cutting Out the Wine (Yes, You Can Whine about It, But It Has Got to Go!)

Much like coffee, alcohol is often seen as a good friend, and we look forward to a glass of wine, beer, or a cocktail at the end of the day. In fact, many people have not gone a day without a glass or two in decades. They might rely on it to "wind down." Also like coffee, there are health benefits to moderate amounts of alcohol. A glass of wine a few times a week has actually been shown to offer protective effects against several diseases including heart disease and cancer. So after the program, moderate consumption of alcohol (approximately three to six drinks per week) is fine, especially organic red wine.

But again, there are numerous downsides, and so taking a short break is a very good idea. Alcohol is high in sugar, taxes the liver, and is a powerful nervous system depressant, which can lead to mood imbalances over time. Prolonged or heavy alcohol use can damage the liver and cause nutrient deficiencies and digestive trouble—including leaky gut and poor absorption. Alcohol depletes magnesium; one likely reason many people suffer from migraines the morning after a few drinks. Heavy alcohol use increases the risk of developing breast and some other cancers, raises our heart disease risk, can lead to liver damage, and also is a mood depressant. Binge drinking can even lead to dangerous cardiac arrhythmias.

Some helpful tips for cutting the alcohol:

- Weaning off gradually and using other ways to reduce stress are important. Taking L-glutamine can help with cravings and repair damage to the gut lining.

- Depending on how much you rely on it, you will want to slowly cut down on the alcohol in phase one, avoid it completely during phase two, and then you may gradually add it back in during phase three when you are ready.

Exercise Smarter

If you are doing a lot of sitting, it is time to get up and move a little bit more. Our bodies are not designed to sit for long periods of time. Doing so wreaks havoc on the metabolism. Remember, every little bit counts—even getting up to get a glass of water, washing the dishes, or bending down to tie your shoes! You don't need to sign up for a gym; just put on some sneakers and hit the sidewalk. If you are not at all active, start slow. Try to get at least ten minutes of moderate exercise at least three days a week. And try not to sit for more than a couple hours at a time ever! If you and your joints are healthy enough to lift weights or do weight-bearing activities, that will help to prevent muscle loss and boost metabolism.

If you are on the other end of the spectrum and have been logging a lot of cardio miles, give yourself permission to take it down a notch or mix it up. Remember, our bodies are just not designed to do cardio exercise for long periods of time. All the pounding in the gym and on the pavement can actually be doing exactly the opposite of what you want: raising your stress hormone cortisol! So during this phase, your exercise regimen should be focused on lowering your cortisol and stress levels, not increasing them. If you are a runner or usually hit the hour-long cardio classes at the gym five days a week, consider swapping out some more healing exercise such as yoga, walking, or short cardio bursts mixed with weight training. If you have an opportunity to walk barefoot or outside in the sunlight, then do so.

Always check with your doctor before beginning any exercise regimen, especially if you plan to do any intense exercise.

Seven Days In: Are You Ready to Move On?

This questionnaire will help you determine if you are ready to transition into phase two.

- ❑ Are you having at least one firm, easy-to-pass bowel movement a day? This is essential before moving on to phase two. If not, review chapter three.

- ❑ Are you drinking enough water to pass urine approximately every three hours? It should be a light lemon yellow color (not clear or dark).

- ❑ Are you falling asleep easily and sleeping well through the night?

- ❑ Are you waking up feeling more refreshed and energized?

- ❑ Have you been able to cut down on your caffeine intake because your energy is more stable?

- ❑ Are you ready to replace your morning cup of coffee with green tea (or get rid of it altogether)?

- ❑ Have you increased your intake of plant-based foods? We want to shoot for filling one-third to one-half of our plate at each meal, so that means approximately six to nine servings daily.

- ❑ Have you broken up with sugar and artificial sweeteners? If so, you might have realized just how sweet plain fruit really is!

- ❑ Have your cravings for sugar, salt, or fat leveled out/diminished? Are you feeling more in control of your appetite and blood sugar?

- ❑ If you have experienced any headaches or muscle aches/pains, are those diminishing or gone?

❏ Are you feeling comfortable with the preparation and planning of the recipes and meals?

❏ Are your moods feeling more balanced and stable?

❏ Are you excited to take it to the next level?

If you answered "yes" to most of the above questions, then you should be ready to move on to phase two! If you answered "no" to more than two or three, it might make sense to stick with phase one for a little while longer. Some people need a little longer to break up with sugar, fix their fats, improve their digestion, and get rid of key trigger foods. Don't feel guilty. Take your time, and move on when you are ready.

❧ 13 ❧

Phase Two
Immersion/Cleanse ReBoot

You've spent the past week or so easing in by increasing your intake of water, healthy fats, and plant-based foods, and you have kicked the sugary, high glycemic foods to the curb. You have also started to remove the top common intolerance foods. Hopefully you are starting to see a positive shift in your digestion, energy, sleep, and weight. Now it is time to take it to the next level and push your progress forward. In this phase, you will immerse yourself in the experience and gently support your body to cleanse. When we eat or drink foods that create toxic loads, over time our metabolism starts acting like a computer that has been programmed wrong. This phase is designed to "reprogram" your system; it can also improve digestion and absorption, mood, hormone balance, metabolism/energy, sleep, skin and hair, brain functioning, and immunity.

In this phase we will:

1. Stop introducing new toxins.

2. Boost the antioxidants and nutrients that we bring into the body.

3. Support the body to guide/usher out existing toxins.

Stop Introducing Toxins

To accomplish this, take another close look at your diet and household goods. If you have not already, remove processed foods that contain chemicals, additives, nitrates, preservatives, excess heavy metals, and artificial flavors, colorings, etc. Avoid laundry and cleaning products with chemicals, avoid nonorganic produce (especially the Dirty Dozen), and choose only organic or grass-fed animal proteins. Consider limiting other sources of toxins as well: cellphone radiation, toxic relationships, too much screen time, etc.

Increase the Antioxidants and Nutrients in the Diet

- Focus on filling one-third to one-half of your plate with plant-based foods at each meal (also shoot for at least 50 percent raw if possible). Daily consumption of fiber-rich plant-based foods serves to nourish, alkalize, and heal the body and draw toxins out.

- Stay hydrated! Soups, smoothies, fresh-pressed juices, and plenty of filtered water—it all adds up!

- Get plenty of healthy fats. These keep hunger hormones in check and help the body absorb nutrients.

- Choose clean, organic animal proteins.

- Strictly limit all forms of sugar, gluten, and other eliminated foods.

Support the Body to Eliminate Toxins

- High-fiber foods and plenty of liquids support a daily bowel movement/elimination.

- Support digestion with fermented foods, probiotics, and aloe vera juice if needed.

- Exercise to a light sweat to excrete toxins (but avoid overdoing it).

Food Elimination in Phase Two

In phase one, you worked to gradually eliminate some foods and drinks. Now, you will strictly avoid the elimination foods for at least seven days and longer if you like.

Foods to strictly avoid:

1. Sugar/artificial sweeteners
2. Wheat/gluten

3. Dairy (except grass-fed ghee)

4. Soy

5. Corn

6. Alcoholic beverages

7. Coffee

8. *Optionally:* eggs (See other optional considerations below.)

Find recipes in chapter sixteen—and more at www.perfect metabolism.com.

Perfect Metabolism Meal Plan

This meal plan provides a general guideline for you to follow this week. The recipes referred to here can be found in chapter sixteen. You may also choose other recipes or create your own meal plan. (You can download a blank meal plan at *www.perfectmetabolism.com* or use the template provided at the back of the book.)

Key Tips for All Day

- Hydrate! Start each morning with a full glass of filtered water (optionally adding lemon juice and/or a small pinch of salt).

- Load up on veggies! Have as many non-starchy veggies as you like.

- Make sure you are getting plenty of *healthy fats* each day/meal/ snack. This is key!

- Leftovers are great, use them to save time the next day.

- Take time for "soul food." Schedule it into your calendar if you need to.

- If you need a snack, go for it—although they are not required. Remember to reach for options that have proteins, healthy fats, and/ or fiber.

- Doing some prep work after dinner helps with digestion and makes tomorrow easier.

- Allow time to settle down each evening before bedtime, avoiding electronics one hour before bed.

- By week two, your blood sugar should ideally be stable enough to allow twelve hours between dinner and breakfast, which may help the body to boost the metabolism and burn fat more effectively.
- Every few days look over the recipes, decide what you want to make, create your shopping list, and shop for what you need.

DAY ONE			
Breakfast	*Lunch*	*Snack*	*Dinner*
Superfood Smoothie of your choice (Include chia seeds and coconut oil if you did not already take it in your tea.)	Big bowl of Power Greens Soup	Almond butter on green apple slices	Wild Salmon with Mustard and Dill Sauce Roasted Broccoli and Cauliflower Quinoa (Make 3x extra! We will use this several times again over the next couple days.)
Record how you are doing, thoughts, feelings, and cravings:			
Evening Prep			
Prep salad ingredients for tomorrow: rinse, dry, and chop if you like. Roast beets if you will be including in the salad. Make salad dressing for tomorrow's lunch.			

DAY TWO

Breakfast	Lunch	Snack	Dinner
Superfood Smoothie of your choice	Salad with Green Goddess Dressing (Make a big salad and be sure to include at least ½ avocado. Include any leftover roasted broccoli/cauliflower or other veggies, and add leftover salmon or chicken or another protein if you like, and toss in some quinoa.)	Quick Pick-Me-Up Drink	Baked chicken topped with Quick Lemon Herb Vinaigrette Baked Mashed Cauliflower "Potatoes" Ratatouille (mixed sautéed veggies) (Make extra of everything!)

Record how you are doing, thoughts, feelings, and cravings:

Evening Prep

Prep Hummus Dip if you are making it for tomorrow. It is a great snack or appetizer.

DAY THREE

Breakfast	Lunch	Snack	Dinner
Frittata or Super-food Smoothie of your choice	Salmon on quinoa (Warm up leftovers from salmon dinner including veggies from last night, or sauté some veggies and toss together with some leftover mustard sauce.) *Optional:* green salad with simple dressing	Hummus Dip or mashed avocado with veggies (peppers, cucumbers, carrot sticks, etc.)	Steak (or grilled chicken or fish) with Chimichurri Sauce Roasted sweet potatoes (½ cup) Lemony Green Beans

Record how you are doing, thoughts, feelings, and cravings:

Evening Prep

Make Mexican Chicken Soup for tomorrow and pesto sauce if you will be using.

DAY FOUR

Breakfast	Lunch	Snack	Dinner
Veggie Egg Scramble with avocado and salsa, or Superfood Smoothie if you are avoiding eggs	Mexican Chicken Soup with avocado and chopped veggies (Make soup the night before or the day before in a slow cooker.)	Quick Pick-Me-Up Drink	Zucchini or spaghetti squash "noodles" topped with a quality jarred marinara sauce or homemade pesto sauce *Optional:* top with organic nitrate-free and preservative-free sausage (bake in oven or sauté)

Record how you are doing, thoughts, feelings, and cravings:

Evening Prep

Soak your cashews and make the Garlic Herbed Cashew Cheese dip if you will be using tomorrow.

If you want, you could make your Chia Pudding for the morning. Set it in the fridge and it will be ready to go when you wake up!

DAY FIVE			
Breakfast	*Lunch*	*Snack*	*Dinner*
Chia Pudding with fresh blueberries, chopped walnuts, and shredded unsweetened coconut	Salad with avocado and pumpkin seeds or nuts (Add in a quarter cup of leftover quinoa if you like and/or leftover chicken.)	Chopped veggies and Garlic Herbed Cashew Cheese dip, or a cup of the soup broth	Mexican Chicken Soup with lots of veggies and avocado chunks (If you need a starchy carb serving, add in a small amount of cooked rice: approx. one-third cup)

Record how you are doing, thoughts, feelings, and cravings:

Evening Prep

Stop at the store to shop for the rest of the week's fresh ingredients.

Make a batch of "Cheesy" Kale Chips.

Frequently Asked Questions

Can I eat out or use recipes that are not included in this book?

Yes! If you want to go out to eat or use other recipes, please do. Just keep the guidelines in mind. If you go to a burger joint, find one that offers grass-fed beef, and have it on a lettuce wrap. The same goes for Mexican food: Want a taco? Get it grilled instead of breaded or fried, and ask for it on a lettuce wrap, or have a bowl with lots of veggies and go light on the rice. You may use your own recipes you find on the Internet or in another cookbook too. Most Paleo recipes fit into the guidelines.

Can I eat fruit?

If you are trying to reset your metabolism and improve your insulin sensitivity, during phase two, ideally restricting yourself to only one or two servings of low-sugar fruits like berries, green apples, citrus fruits, dragon fruit, and acai berries will be your best bet. A small section of a frozen banana (not too ripe) can count as a serving for smoothies—to thicken them and add natural sweetness. No fruit juice is allowed since these have no fiber and will spike your blood sugar and stimulate your appetite. I would also avoid dried fruits, even though they have natural sugars, because these are very concentrated sources of sugar and some contain sulfites as well.

Can I eat things like red meat?

What we are trying to do is break free from the carb and sugar cycle, and protein is an important helper in leveling out blood sugar. So many of us have been told that saturated fats and foods like steak and bacon are bad for our health. But new research is showing this is not true (as long as you use organic/pastured or grass-fed and nitrate-free sources, which are naturally higher in omega-3s and not given antibiotics or growth hormones). So you *can* eat things like steak or even a hamburger—just served on a lettuce wrap instead of a bun. (And don't douse it in ketchup, just stick with low-sugar Dijon mustard.) You can even have bacon on this plan as long as it is nitrate-free/organic. But during phase two, you might choose to avoid beef and bacon because they are a little harder on the digestion. Keep portion sizes for animal proteins about the size of your palm or a deck of playing cards. Too much protein can be acidifying to the body.

Can I buy bottled salad dressings?

The majority of bottled salad dressings contain industrial oils like soy, sugars, or HFCS—all stuff we want to avoid. Some even have sugar listed as the first ingredient! So I recommend sticking with the recipes in this book or making a nice simple dressing right in your salad bowl just using olive or avocado oil, lemon juice and/or vinegar, herbs and salt/pepper. However, one store-bought dressing that I like is Tessemae's (*www.tessemaes .com*) which uses olive oil and can be found at Whole Foods.

Can the whole family do this program?

This program is not designed for kids. But getting kids to cut down on super sweet foods and drinks for a little while can be a great thing for their immunity, moods, digestion, etc. If you are getting kids involved, I recommend modifying the program for them to mainly focus on getting **processed foods and sugars out** (the candies, sodas, sweets, etc.). One great goal with kids is to increase the plant-based foods they eat. Kids should be able to eat any and all whole fruits as something sweet in place of a sugary snack or treat, but it is a good idea to cut out the fruit juice for the week. Juice spikes blood sugar and stimulates appetite. Most kids also love smoothies, but they might prefer the recipes just slightly sweeter than the way they are here (i.e., replace some of the plain water with more coconut water, or you could add a little bit more banana or fruit or add a teaspoon of coconut palm nectar or honey if desired). If you add coconut oil, protein powder, or chia seeds to their smoothie, use one-quarter to one-half the recommended amounts in the recipes.

Is this a low-carb diet? Will I have enough energy?

The majority of carbs in this program should could from nutritious slow carbohydrates like vegetables, nuts, certain whole fruits, low glycemic starches like sweet potatoes, and if you like one or two servings of non-gluten grains each day. If you are finding that you do not have the energy you need to go about your day, you might choose to add an additional serving of carbohydrates in the evening, or increase your coconut oil intake in the morning. If you are training very hard or working out for long periods, you might want to restart this program when you can cut your activity levels down or move more gradually into the program.

It is possible to experience some fatigue and headaches, which could be an indicator of some die-off effect (release of toxins). Serious fatigue or headaches could mean that there is an overgrowth of candida, and you might need more support for moving forward. (Please contact your doctor if you are experiencing any issues.)

I really enjoy my workouts, and I do sweat a lot. I'm concerned I won't have enough to eat especially before my workout.

Depending on your adrenal health, you might want to cut back on your cardio for a little while. But if you are up for being more active, you might need to adjust the amounts and types of foods you eat from day to day. If you are working out, you might need an additional serving of carbs, protein, and/or fat. Sweating is good for removing toxins from the body. Have an orange or apple, and a handful of nuts or a piece of fruit before breakfast—or a few minutes before your workout. But there also might be days when you are feeling a little lethargic or tired. On those days, choosing a gentler exercise like walking or yoga might feel better. Remember, exercising harder is not always better, because it can raise our stress hormones!

Is it normal to have a headache? Can I take ibuprofen?

Sometimes, when we remove toxins from the body, we can have a few days when we feel worse before we feel better. Make sure your digestion is moving and you are getting plenty of fluids and fiber. Headaches can be a common symptom of cutting down on caffeine as well. I like to use homeopathic pain remedies (many natural stores carry them). Also, dill, turmeric, and magnesium can help with headaches. But if you have any debilitating headaches or other concerning health issues, please stop the program and consult a medical doctor if they do not improve.

I am a big gum chewer—do I have to give that up? I find that if I don't chew gum, I eat more, so I am worried about stopping.

Gum chewing is not recommended on this program. Most gum contains ingredients that we are trying to avoid because they can interfere with our metabolism and digestion, including petroleum and artificial sweeteners, colors, and flavors. If you must have gum, choose a natural brand that does not have artificial ingredients. Still, most contain xylitol, which in some people or in large amounts can be troublesome for the digestion.

I'm worried about giving up sugar. I have tried to in the past and failed. Do you have any tips to help with this?

The first three to four days of giving up sugar are usually the hardest. Many of us have a certain time of day when we crave sugar. Drink Golden Milk Tea or an herbal tea with a spoonful of coconut oil at that time, take a short walk, or do some of the prep work in the kitchen for the next day instead. Making sure you are getting enough healthy fats in your diet is key. Review chapter one for some other recommendations for supporting yourself in breaking up with sugar.

The cool thing about giving up sugar is once you go a week or two, you can essentially change your taste buds. Many of the things that used to taste yummy will seem sickly sweet after the break, and therefore you can really "lose" your sweet tooth. So keep your eye on that prize! Just remind yourself that getting sugar out of your diet is perhaps one of the best things you can do because sugar:

- Makes us hungrier
- Ages us from the inside out (by creating advance glycation end products, which damage collagen and elastin)
- Causes oxidation of cells, which also lowers our immunity
- Promotes candida overgrowth, inflammation, and adrenal fatigue
- Creates insulin resistance, which many people do not know they have, which is a diabetes precursor and also causes stubborn weight gain
- Makes us tired and moody
- Raises our risk of all diseases (heart disease, diabetes, cancers).

Visit *www.perfectmetabolism.com* to see more FAQs or to submit your own question.

What If I Am Not Feeling Energized or Great?

One reason that you might not be feeling great is that your body is still not eliminating toxins efficiently. You might want to consider adding herbs or supplements to support your detox. Milk thistle, artichoke, or dandelion can support the liver. Vitamin C can also support the body to detoxify, ideally from a whole food source such as camu camu or acerola cherry. Sweating is another very effective way to get toxins out of the body, either from exercise or in a sauna. Make sure to stay well-hydrated all day long; this is extremely important.

Perhaps you could be experiencing an intolerance to a food that you have not eliminated. Although quite effective, a food elimination diet is not 100 percent foolproof. It is limited to the foods that you remove, and it is also somewhat subjective. People can be intolerant to almost any food. You might need to consider removing other foods or having a food intolerance panel run.

Other eliminations to consider if the following areas are not improving:

- ⚜ Arthritis or joint pain? Consider cutting nightshades, which include potatoes, tomatoes, bell/hot peppers, eggplant, and tomatillos.

- ⚜ Thyroid trouble? Consider taking out raw goitrogenic foods—cruciferous vegetables (bok choy, broccoli, brussels sprouts, cabbage, cauliflower, kale, spinach), peaches, peanuts, pine nuts, radishes, strawberries, soy, turnips.

- ⚜ Irritable bowel syndrome? Remove the FODMAPs—short-chain carbohydrates high in fructose, fructans, and polyols, including onion, garlic, watermelon, apple, breads, sugar alcohols, fructose, beet, and avocado. (You can find a full list of FODMAPs online.) FODMAPs tend to ferment in the gut, which can lead to gas, pain, diarrhea, and bloating. After you remove FODMAPs, the bacterial balance of the gut needs to be addressed. Often IBS is caused by an overgrowth of bacteria in the small intestine (SIBO).

- ⚜ Other possible underlying issues that could be causing you to not feel your best include a parasite or viral infection, adrenal fatigue, candida overgrowth, heavy metal toxicity, hypothyroidism, or other issues. If you have not done so already, schedule an appointment with an integrative doctor or health practitioner who can help you figure out what is happening in your particular case.

Key Tips for Each Day

- ⚜ Within twenty minutes of getting up, have an eight-ounce glass of filtered water. *Optional:* Add the juice of half a lemon and a pinch of high-quality salt. Stay hydrated throughout the day with water, soups, smoothies, and plant-based foods.

- ⚜ Try to allow twelve hours between dinner and breakfast to help boost the metabolism and burn fat more effectively. Ideally, eat dinner before 7 p.m., and no snacking afterward. If you get enough fat at dinner and your blood sugar is stable, you should be able to go twelve hours.

- Strive to fill half your plate with organic plant-based foods. Load up on veggies!

- Follow the Rule of Three: get healthy fats, fiber, and/or protein at each meal/snack.

- Snack smart. reach for plant-based foods, proteins, or nuts before carbs.

- Take time for "soul food." Schedule it on your calendar if you need to.

- Instead of plopping down on the couch right after dinner, take a short walk or make time to do some prep work for the next day. It helps with digestion and makes tomorrow easier. Studies show that people who do the dishes tend to be a healthier weight!

- Give yourself time to settle down each evening before bedtime. Ideally, say no TV in bed and no electronics one hour before bed.

Are You Ready to Move On?

Some people might be feeling so great during this phase that they choose to carry on for another seven days or longer! That is up to you. You can hold out in this phase as long as you are enjoying it. When you are ready to find out if you are sensitive to the foods you have eliminated, you are ready to step into phase three.

❧ 14 ❧

Phase Three
ReIntroduce

Congratulations for making it to phase three! Now it is time to isolate which foods might be tipping your metabolism out of balance. To do this, we will *challenge* the eliminated foods by reintroducing them one at a time. It is important not to rush through this stage, because it might interfere with your ability to clearly link a reaction to a particular food. It can also overwhelm the body to restore eliminated foods and substances too quickly. So be gentle with yourself.

You'll want to wait at least twenty-four to forty-eight hours between each food because sometimes reactions can take a day or more to appear. Keep in mind that many different systems in the body can be affected by food intolerances: digestive, neurological, respiratory, mental health, energy, sleep, etc.

How will you know if you are sensitive to a food? Although it is not always clear, here are some of the common signs and symptoms. Some will show up almost immediately; others will take several hours or longer:

- Stuffy or runny nose and/or sinus pain/pressure
- A feeling of something stuck in the throat, needing to clear the throat
- Headaches/migraines
- Coughing or sneezing (often repeatedly)
- Digestive trouble—gas, reflux, pain, bloating, diarrhea, constipation, discomfort
- Foggy thinking, poor focus, or memory issues
- Fatigue, lethargy, sleepiness

- ⚘ Mood imbalances—depression, sadness, more emotional, anger, anxiety

- ⚘ Joint pain or muscle aches

- ⚘ An itchy nose, mouth, or other areas of skin

- ⚘ Rashes or other skin conditions, such as acne

- ⚘ Racing pulse—this is actually one way to diagnose food intolerances. If your pulse quickens after eating something, you could be intolerant to that food.

Because symptoms may not arise if you only eat a small amount of the food, have more than one serving of the challenge food on the day that you reintroduce it. *But if you get symptoms right away from a single serving, it is not necessary to eat it again!*

When we come to this phase, people often say, "Do I *have* to reintroduce gluten (or dairy or soy)?" The answer is no, you certainly do not. If you feel so much better without a certain food that you do not wish to reintroduce it, don't! You do not have to challenge a food if you do not wish to. Or you can stay off it for a longer period of time and decide to challenge it later. This is totally up to you.

Foods to Reintroduce in Phase Three

1. **Eggs.** If you removed eggs, they are one of the first foods to bring back. Why? Because they are so good for us, and if you have no problems with them, I want you to be able to include them in your diet! Eggs are an excellent source of protein (6.3 grams each) and contain choline, tryptophan, and selenium—all very good for our health. As with all animal proteins, it is worth every penny to buy organic eggs, even better if you can get the pasture-raised kind. People sometimes react to the GMO feed given to conventional hens, and going with non-GMO organic eggs is all they need to eliminate the problem. The whites contain the majority of the protein, but one of the most nutritious parts of the egg is the yolk; it contains the choline, omega-3s, and other important nutrients. So eat the yolks! If you are paying extra for pastured eggs, you will see how orange the yolks are—that is the extra omega-3s and other nutrients!

Eat a breakfast of eggs, and see if any symptoms crop up over the next day or so. You could have something made with eggs again later in the day. Try to eat eggs more than once on your challenge day. Write down any symptoms. If no symptoms arise within 48 hours, then you are likely not sensitive to eggs.

2. **Coffee.** *Ahhhh, coffee.* Some people might be missing it a lot, others might be pleasantly surprised that they are able to function without it and are not sure they even need it. The main drawbacks to drinking coffee are it delivers a jolt of caffeine (cortisol spike) and it is dehydrating and acidifying. If you wish to return to coffee, consider drinking half caffeinated (the other half should be Swiss Water Processed decaf) and choosing a low-acid brand (or you can add pH drops to your coffee cup). This will help to lessen the caffeine jolt and lower the acidity. Be sure to drink a full glass of water before your cup o' joe, and another one not too long after. Also I hate to say it, but the sweetener needs to go! It stimulates your sweet tooth. And whatever you do, do not use those powdered creamers, which are little packets of trans fats! I would rather you use organic cream (if you can tolerate dairy) or unsweetened coconut or cashew cream. Add a teaspoon of coconut oil into your coffee to boost the metabolism and keep hunger hormones in check. Also, make sure to get plenty of foods rich in B vitamins and magnesium if you return to coffee (caffeine dumps these nutrients).

   Stay mindful: if you do go back to coffee and find that you are quickly back up to more than two cups a day, consider scaling back again.

3. **Dairy.** It is estimated that only about 40 percent of the population has the ability to digest the lactose in milk. Some people find that they can tolerate goat's milk better than cow's milk. Staying organic is key for milk. Milk from cows not raised on organic feed is associated with an increased risk of several types of cancer.

   If you react to dairy, you could be reacting to the casein, whey, or lactose.

Take your time and try introducing several different types of dairy to see how your body responds. Here are a few options to consider:

◆ Start with grass-fed butter first. Even if you can't handle cow's milk, you might tolerate butter. Grass-fed butter is a stable, delicious, and wonderful fat.

◆ Next up, goat's or sheep's milk. Goat's milk does not contain agglutinin, so it is significantly easier to digest than cow's milk.

◆ Raw cow's milk may be tolerated better because it has not been pasteurized and contains the enzymes needed for lactose digestion. Some people might find that milk from grass-fed Jersey cows, which contain the A2 casein (not the A1 Holstein variety, which the majority of milk comes from) is a better option.

◆ Next up is yogurt. Because it is fermented, yogurt may be better tolerated (just avoid the kind with lots of added sugars or artificial sweeteners).

◆ By all means, **skip the skim and low-fat options for any and all dairy!** Yes, if you are able to tolerate dairy, go for the full fat. Remember that fats are critical for hunger control and overall health. Plus, according to Sally Fallon, author of the popular cookbook *Nourishing Traditions*, powdered milk is added to reduced-fat dairy products, which adds damaged and oxidized proteins. Skim and reduced-fat varieties are also higher in sugar. Studies support it: people who drink full-fat milk are more likely to be a healthy weight than those who drink low-fat or skim milk.

4. **Corn.** When reintroducing corn, always look for non-GMO or organic corn. Even better if you can find it is sprouted corn, which further improves the nutrition and digestibility of corn and other grains. If you find that you are not sensitive to corn, I recommend always choosing organic or non-GMO and limiting it to two to three servings per week total.

5. **Wine/alcohol.** If you were able to give up wine and beer during the program, bravo! This is one of the hardest things for many people to do because it is such a surefire way to decompress

at the end of a stressful day. It can make us more social and relaxed. If you tried but were not able to give it up, then I highly recommend that you pick up *The Mood Cure* by Julia Ross.

When reintroducing alcoholic beverages, make sure you take it slow. Realize that alcohol can contain gluten grains (beer and some spirits), tannins, and sulfites. You could be reacting to any of those things. If you react to wine, you might find that you do better with organic wine, because it has fewer sulfites and tannins. Because (most) beer contains gluten, reintroducing beer should come with reintroducing gluten, unless you choose a gluten-free variety. Some beers also contain high fructose corn syrup. When you reintroduce alcohol, I suggest starting with just one glass and having it with a meal to minimize its impact on your body. Moderate consumption of alcohol (one glass for women, two for men)—especially red wine—has been shown to lower the risk of breast cancer and heart disease. But drinking more than one glass for women (two for men) raises our risk of many diseases and can strain an already overtaxed liver. Moderation is absolutely key with alcohol.

Foods You Might Just Want to Live Without

1. **Wheat.** Because just one serving of wheat or gluten can cause damage to the gut lining, this is one food type that you might decide that you just don't need to reintroduce. Neither wheat nor gluten contains any essential nutrients that we cannot obtain from other foods. You'll recall that one of the reasons we are seeing a rise in wheat and gluten allergies and sensitivities is because it is hybridized and highly processed and has (sometimes lots of) extra gluten added to it. If you wish to reintroduce wheat, start with something that is minimally processed (last time I saw the ingredients on a typical supermarket wheat bread, I was shocked at how processed it is). Start with sprouted organic wheat or a traditional sourdough (fermented wheat) that does not have any added gluten on the list of ingredients. Another option is to choose an ancient form of wheat, like einkorn, which some people can tolerate better than modern

wheat. When reintroducing wheat, give it at least a couple of days before reintroducing another food, as the reaction can be delayed and very subtle. Just remember that most conventional wheat breads are about as far from healthy as you can get with lots of added ingredients that you do not need—like dough conditioners and high fructose corn syrup.

2. **Gluten.** This does what its name suggests: it provides the "glue" that gives breads that soft springy feel. In addition to being naturally part of wheat and other grains, gluten is added to many products. Because no one can fully digest gluten proteins, it could potentially be damaging everyone's guts. Some of us just might not know about it yet. If you do not notice a reaction to gluten but choose to reintroduce it, I still recommend limiting it as much as possible. *Note: Whatever you do, if for any reason you think you might have celiac disease, do not reintroduce wheat or gluten. Please see your doctor to be tested first. People with celiac disease must avoid all forms of gluten completely and should not ever challenge it.*

3. **Soy.** Found in many processed foods, salad dressings, mayonnaise, cereals, sports bars, and protein powders, soy is something you might have been unknowingly consuming. Again, most soy is GMO, has a high amount of phytic acid, which can rob the body of nutrients, and is poorly digested. The only way to remove the phytic acids is fermentation, so organic fermented is the only form of soy that should be consumed regularly. Miso is an example of fermented soy, so miso soup is a nice way to introduce soy back in. If you do tolerate soy, would an occasional edamame hurt you? No, I personally have a few whenever I eat sushi, and a little tofu in my miso soup about once a month. But I totally avoid any highly processed soy, including soy milk, soy protein bars and shakes, and any other fake meat product that is made with soy.

Foods That I Do Not Recommend Reintroducing

1. **High fructose corn syrup, candy, sweets.** You might be pleasantly surprised to find that sweetened foods and drinks that you used to enjoy taste sickly sugary to you now. When we give

up sugar and sweetened foods for a period of time, we can reset not only our metabolism, but also our taste buds. Remember, it is not possible to have a healthy metabolism and stay a healthy weight if your blood sugar is not under control. Limiting sweetened foods/drinks is one of the best things you can do for your health, weight, energy, and disease prevention. You went to a lot of trouble getting them out of your diet, so why reintroduce nutrient-devoid super sweet processed foods at all? If you do choose to occasionally sweeten your foods, stick with the natural sweeteners and keep it to less than 5 percent of your total calorie intake or six teaspoons of added sugars daily—whichever is less.

2. **Highly processed/packaged foods.** Especially avoid anything with chemicals, artificial colors, preservatives—the fewer of these foods we consume, the better. Remember that toxins tell our bodies to store fat! Realize that not all foods that come in a bag or box are bad; just make sure to read the label and know what you are spending your money and your health on!

3. **Processed table salt.** This is an easy one because you can just replace with Himalayan pink salt, Celtic gray salt, or unprocessed sea salt. Processed table salt is great for science experiments and to melt snow, but not to eat.

4. **Sodas: both diet and regular.** If you can stay off sodas, that is ideal. Sodas provide zero nutrition, contribute to weight gain (both diet and regular), raise our risk of diabetes, and heart disease, and some research shows that regular consumption interferes with memory and learning. Sodas also contain phosphorus, which in excess is bad for our bones. I used to drink lots of them, and instead I now enjoy kombucha tea, unsweetened iced tea with lemon, or an occasional sparkling water.

What If I Had a Reaction? Do I Need to Avoid That Food Forever?

If you reacted to a food, it does not *necessarily* mean you will react to it forever. Only time will tell. If you react to a food, you should remove that food from your diet again, and ideally strictly avoid it for a period of about three to six months, depending on how severe the reaction was or how much of a staple it was in your diet. Foods that you reacted more severely to or that you used to eat more frequently should be removed for longer. In the meantime, you will want to heal the gut. Taking a high-quality probiotic is important. Bone broths and gut repair supplements like L-glutamine can also support the healing of the mucosal barrier. Because gut inflammation is often at the root of food intolerances, avoiding the food and healing the gut will make it more likely for you to tolerate that food again. At the end of the longer elimination, you can reintroduce that food again to see if there is a reaction. Some foods you might always react to, and these should ideally be avoided forever. If you can tolerate a food again, it is important to not eat it too often because you could end up right back where you started. Place that food on a rotation diet where you eat it no more than once every four days.

Are You Ready to Move On?

If you have reintroduced all the eliminated foods that you wish to enjoy again and are clear about which ones (if any) are causing you trouble, you are ready to move on to phase four where you take what you have learned from this program and merge it with real life to find your forever Perfect Metabolism plan.

❧ 15 ❧

Phase Four
ReNew—Merge/Move On

*C*ongrats *on completing the Perfect Metabolism Plan! That is an amazing achievement!* Hopefully you are thriving from your diet rich in plant-based foods, healthy fats, and grass-fed proteins. Perhaps your cravings have diminished, you are sleeping better, feeling more energized and less stress, and your weight is more balanced. Maybe you have even found some answers to your perplexing health problem right at the end of your fork. Above all, I hope you have learned a lot through this process and are feeling renewed, because . . .

Knowledge Is Power

One of my clients said that embarking on the Perfect Metabolism Plan made her feel "powerful." This was especially profound coming from her as a breast cancer survivor. I agree with her: it is very empowering to be more on top of your health, especially if you have ever felt like it was spiraling out of control. We know what out-of-control stress can do to our metabolism and health!

Food may not always be the answer to every health issue. But I think Ann Wigmore said it best:

> *The food you eat can be either the safest and most powerful form of medicine or the slowest form of poison.*

Do I Have to Be Perfect to Have a Perfect Metabolism?

A lot of people often wonder at this stage: How close do I have to stick to the principles to keep my metabolism working optimally? In other words, *"Do I have to be perfect to have a perfect metabolism?"* Can I enjoy an occasional bowl of gelato or go for hamburgers and fries? Ha! That might be the million-dollar question, right? The answer is, it depends.

The 90/10 Rule

Author, teacher, and naturopath Steven Schechter, who is head of the Natural Healing Institute said something in a class that always stuck with me: "It is the things that we do most of the time that have the biggest impact on our health."

So if we eat ice cream every night, it is going to impact our health more than if we indulge in it once or twice a month. If we take chia seeds or coconut oil every day, it will have a bigger impact on our health than if we take them every now and then or "if we remember to." Eating lots of vegetables every day will impact our health much more than a small serving of overcooked peas shoved to the side of our dinner plate once or twice a week.

The 90/10 rule gives you a little (but not too much) wiggle room. It is not always easy to do something 100 percent every single day of the year. So if 90 percent of our day, week, and month is filled with the ideal healthy choices and only 10 percent is left for splurge foods or less ideal choices, then you and your metabolism are more likely to stay balanced. I tend to feel my very best when I am closer to 95 and 5 percent, but there are times I might stray closer to 85 percent healthy choices/15 percent splurges—such as on vacation.

Because each of us is unique, some might be able to stray farther than others and keep those dominoes from crashing down. Others will have less leeway. Hopefully if you have made these powerful changes to your metabolism, you have some pretty powerful incentives to stay on this good path. But I know that *life happens.* We get busy, have to travel, deadlines loom, and we fall prey to temptations or stress. We might not have the time or inspiration to make home-cooked meals every day. *I experience all those challenges too!* Want to hear the ultimate irony? While writing this book, I gained a couple of pounds! Yep, I know! I was writing about all the things you need to know to keep your metabolism humming along, but I wasn't *doing* all those things. I was doing some things that are not good for the metabolism—sitting too much, stressing about deadlines and details, spending too much time in front of screens, not sleeping enough, all while trying to uphold commitments and support my family and clients. Those few pounds were just one symptom that my metabolism and health were tipping out of balance. I also wasn't sleeping quite as well. But thankfully, as soon as I could, I put myself and my health back up on top of my priority list, got moving again, lowered my stress levels, put my sleep back on track, and quickly lost those couple pounds. And it was interesting that they had gone right to my midsection (where stress likes to put them)! It is important to remember to keep our health high up on our priority list if we don't want it to spiral totally out of control.

Just remember that if you do find yourself out of balance and back on that hamster wheel, or sugar roller coaster, sitting too much, or not hydrating well, simply return to the principles for a few days to a week and get back on track. You have the tools now to take back your control!

Here are sixteen tips to guide you as you move forward.

16 Perfect Metabolism Tips

1. **Follow the Rule of Three.** Each time you eat, try to get one or more fat, protein, and/or fiber to keep your blood sugar leveled out.

2. **Fat is your friend.** You need plenty of healthy fat every day, or you will crave more sugar and junk food.

3. **Sugar is not your friend.** Use the 5 percent rule with sugar and other indulgences. If you want to indulge, then let it be no more than 5 percent of your total daily calorie intake or about six teaspoons for women.

4. **Avoid foods you are sensitive to.** This seems so obvious, but it is easier said than done. These foods can be tempting. Just remember that eating foods we are intolerant to increases inflammation, can cause many chronic painful symptoms, and can lead to weight gain. And because they can also be addictive, "moderation" is not likely possible.

5. **Be mindful.** Think before you eat: Am I really hungry? Do I really want this? Will it contribute to or take away from my Perfect Metabolism? Even if you know it might take away from it, but you choose to eat it anyway, then sit down, slow down, and really enjoy it!

6. **Plant-based foods can save your life.** Shoot for 9 servings of plant based foods a day—at least!

7. **Do not multitask when eating.** That means no cellphones, computers, TV, or driving. Enjoy your food and the company you are eating with.

8. **Hydrate.** Start each morning with a full glass of water (I like to add fresh lemon), and try to drink half your weight in ounces of water by the end of the day.

9. **Never drink alcohol on an empty stomach.** Limit yourself to one drink per day (two for men), and your metabolism and liver will thank you!

10. **Eat real foods.** Eating plenty of real, clean, fresh foods is very important to metabolism and overall health. Cut the chemicals, flavorings, and fake stuff. If you do choose convenience foods, go for the upgraded version!

11. **Plan ahead.** Planning is key to getting home-cooked meals on the table.

12. **Don't sit too long!** Sitting literally turns off your metabolism. Incorporate lots of little movements all day long, mix in a few intense movements and some weight-bearing ones, and you will be good to go! A short walk after dinner supports digestion, mood, and metabolism.

13. **Get your soul food.** Laugh, have fun, volunteer, take time to do things that make you feel wonderful. When your soul is full, you need to feed your belly less.

14. **Get your beauty sleep.** That is where our recovery happens. Lack of sleep makes us hungrier. Settle down for a good night's rest by turning off electronics an hour before you want to fall asleep.

15. **Listen to your body.** If your body is talking to you, it is rude to ignore it or shut it up with an Advil. Be mindful about how foods make you feel and function. If you do end up veering off course, don't let guilt take over. Connect to your body and to how that choice made you feel, and get back on track.

16. **Demand more from your food.** Food should taste good, but that is simply not enough. When sitting down to eat, consider if that food in front of you will nourish or take away from your health. How will that food affect your body and mind in ten minutes, two hours, the next day, and beyond?

Choose Health

So now it's up to you to find that place where you can *live* in the real world and still *thrive* in your health. Life is full of choices every day, all day long. So now each and every day going forward, you will be faced with a choice:

- ❧ Go back to your old ways of eating and end up right back with that laundry list of symptoms?
- ❧ Choose health?

I hope *most of the time* you choose health! Because you deserve it. You are worth it.

The next chapter contains some delicious recipes for you to use to implement the Perfect Metabolism Plan—enjoy!

❦ 16 ❧

The Perfect Metabolism Recipes

True healthcare reform starts in your kitchen, not in Washington.

—ANONYMOUS

These recipes can be used during the Perfect Metabolism program and as part of your forever plan. I hope that they become new staples! Many of these are family friendly and great as leftovers too!

You may also use your own recipes or find other options online and in cookbooks. You can even go out to eat. Just stick to the ten Perfect Metabolism keys—avoid the foods that have been eliminated, choose the healthy fats (this is a little more difficult to control when eating out, because most restaurants use cheap cooking oils, so keep that in mind), go organic and grass-fed for proteins, use organic produce (at least for the dirty dozen), and kick the sweets to the curb!

Some helpful equipment:

- **Vitamix, Blendtec, or another high-powered emulsifying blender.** If you do not have a really good blender, this is the number-one product I recommend investing in! I burned out the motor on three of the less expensive blenders before I broke down and got my Vitamix. It has been worth every penny.

- **Food processor.** These are great for making pestos, homemade dressings, chopping herbs, etc.

- **Juicer.** I like the "slow" or masticating juicers the best, as they do not generate any heat and preserve the most nutrients.

- **Spiral slicer.** This tool comes in handy for making zucchini pasta and spiral slicing other veggies.

- **Quality, nontoxic pans.** The old Teflon pans are a health hazard. If you still have some around, especially if they are scratched, please replace/upgrade them. It is worth the investment to "go green" with your pans. Look for stainless steel, ceramic, or cast iron, and if you are going to choose a nonstick variety, look for one with no PFOAs. Avoid using metal utensils to prevent scratching the pan's surface.

Plan Ahead Tips

One of the biggest obstacles to successfully maintaining a healthy diet is lack of planning. A little planning goes a long way and can keep you from feeling overwhelmed. Here are some tips:

- Sit down every few days to figure out your meal plan.
- Soak nuts every few days to make your homemade nut milks. (I like to make small batches so they are fresh.)
- If you know you won't have time to cook later, plan to use your slow cooker in the morning.
- If you know that you will need to eat out, do a little research to find some places that offer organic proteins, salads, and gluten-free or grain-free options.
- Have your complete shopping list in hand when you go to the store.
- Set aside some time for cooking things ahead.
- When you make proteins and other things that take longer to cook, prepare extra so you have enough for another meal! For example, cooked chicken or quinoa makes great leftovers in salads.
- Make extra salad for another meal (just do not put dressing on it, or it will get soggy).
- When you are in the kitchen preparing something, maximize your time by making something else (i.e., soak beans, put nuts in water to soak for nut milk, prepare a pesto for tomorrow's dinner, or chop up ingredients for your salad for the next day when you are already making dinner).

- When I make homemade cashew milk, I first get it thick and remove some to use as "cheese," which I season separately. I add more water to the remainder for the cashew cream and/or milk.

- When I make the soup broth, I like to store some in the refrigerator, some in freezer. That way I have some on hand when I need it.

- Make your chia pudding and put it into fridge before you go to bed. It makes a great grab 'n' go snack or breakfast!

- Wash your greens and veggies (dry them thoroughly) before you put them away in the fridge, so they are ready when you need them. You might even want to slice/chop some ahead of time.

- Chop extra fresh herbs, so you have some for the next day. You can even freeze them!

Breakfast

Superfood Smoothies

Superfood smoothies are a great breakfast, or a pre- or post-workout snack. I have a smoothie for breakfast most mornings. Often people say to me: "Smoothies are not enough to keep me going all morning." A smoothie that has a lot of fruit and/or juice can easily make you crash and burn. So to craft a more satisfying smoothie and avoid the sugar roller coaster, skip the fruit juice, keep the fruit to a minimum, and make sure to include healthy fat, fiber, and/or protein (the Rule of Three). Also avoid sweet toppings like granola or added sugars. Sprinkling a good dose of cinnamon in there is another way to support healthy blood sugar.

Do boost your smoothies with superfoods like leafy greens (kale, spinach), greens powders, chia seeds, hemp seeds, flax meal, plant-based protein powder (like hemp or pea protein), maca powder, or coconut oil/butter. Want to know a little trick? I always add in a small pinch of high-quality Himalayan salt to my smoothies—it brings out the sweetness and flavors and boosts the mineral content.

Smoothie Directions
1. Put the liquid in the blender and add chia seeds. Allow them to soak for 3–5 minutes.

2. Put everything else into the blender except any ice and frozen fruit.

3. Blend to combine well.

4. Add frozen fruit (if using) and ice, blend well.

5. Serve immediately.

Antiaging Purple Superfood Smoothie

This is my breakfast most days of the week. It is quick and easy to make—and delicious and energizing too. When I put in the coconut oil and chia seeds, I am satisfied until lunch. Otherwise, I would be hungry within an hour or two.

Ingredients

½ cup filtered water

½ cup coconut water (or nondairy milk like cashew, almond, or coconut)

¼–½ cup frozen wild organic blueberries

2- to 3-inch piece frozen banana (optional but makes smoothie sweeter and thicker)

2 tablespoons chia seeds (soaked)

½ scoop vanilla plant-based protein powder (optional)

1 large handful power greens, baby spinach, or 1 scoop of greens powder

1 teaspoon virgin coconut oil or raw coconut (optional)

1 small pinch Himalayan salt *(brings out the flavors and sweetness)*

Ice as desired to thicken

SuperGreen Smoothie

Ingredients

½ cup filtered water

½ cup coconut water (or nondairy milk like cashew, almond, or coconut)

¼ cup frozen pineapple

2 tablespoons chia seeds

1 big handful dark leafy greens (like baby spinach) or a scoop of greens powder

Ice as desired to thicken

½–1 scoop plant-based (such as Warrior Blend) protein powder

Small pinch pink Himalayan salt

Raw honey, coconut nectar, and/or stevia to taste

Superfood Cacao Smoothie

Ingredients

½ cup coconut water (or nondairy milk like cashew, almond, or coconut)

½ cup water or unsweetened nondairy milk

2 tablespoons unsweetened raw cacao powder

⅓ frozen banana (optional)

Handful dark leafy greens or 1 teaspoon greens powder

2 tablespoons chia seeds (soaked)

½–1 scoop vanilla or chocolate protein powder

1 small pinch Himalayan salt

Ice as desired to thicken

2 teaspoons almond butter (optional)

Pumpkin Cacao Chip Smoothie

Ingredients

¾–1 cup cashew or almond milk (or another alternative milk)

⅓ cup prepared (cooked fresh or canned) pumpkin puree (not pie mix)

½ frozen banana (optional)

2 tablespoons almond butter

2 tablespoons chia seeds

1 scoop vanilla protein powder

Pinch Himalayan salt

Ice as needed to thicken

Raw cacao nibs to top (optional, but adds antioxidants, a nutty dark chocolate taste, and crunch)

Cinnamon is also a delicious addition to consider!

Veggie Egg Scramble

If you are keeping eggs in your diet, scrambles are a great high-protein breakfast and also a great way to get veggies onto your morning plate. I like to lightly sauté veggies (cook the mushrooms, peppers, onions first, they take longer, then add the spinach at the end—use whatever veggies you like, load them up) in coconut oil or ghee, and then crack some eggs into the pan. Cook them over easy or make a scramble, adding salt and pepper to taste. If I want an omelet, I whip up the eggs ahead of time with a little water.

This is also a great way to use up leftover veggies from dinner the night before. Just reheat them in the pan and add the eggs! A sliced avocado is great alongside. I find this to be a delicious lunch too, and I have it often! Another option is to warm up some black beans and have some salsa on the side. If you are eliminating eggs, save these ideas for when you reintroduce them in phase three! Don't overcook the eggs. If you can leave the yolk a little runny, you can avoid destroying some of the nutrients and oxidizing the cholesterol in the egg.

Chia Pudding

Chia seeds soak up liquid and become soft. This energizing breakfast or snack is kind of a like a tapioca pudding—but with tons of omega-3s!

Ingredients

3 tablespoons whole chia seeds

Pinch Himalayan salt

½ teaspoon vanilla powder or extract (and/or cinnamon)

¾–1 cup cashew, coconut, or almond milk (see recipes)

¼ cup fresh or frozen organic blueberries or another berry

2 tablespoons chopped walnuts or hemp hearts

Raw honey, coconut nectar, and/or stevia to taste (optional; start with less, you might not need it at all!)

Directions

1. Stir chia seeds, salt, and vanilla into the milk.
2. Put in refrigerator for 10 minutes up to overnight.
3. Top with blueberries, nuts, hemp hearts, and a few drops of stevia or a light drizzle of the honey or coconut nectar (if using) to serve.

Options

If you would like to serve it warm, warm up the milk in a saucepan, take off heat, stir in chia seeds, and allow to sit and soak up milk for 3–5 minutes. Top with cinnamon and nuts or hemp hearts to serve. Great for breakfast, a snack, or dessert!

Make ahead idea: Put all the ingredients in a glass container before bed, give it a stir, cover, and put into the refrigerator. It will be ready in the morning for breakfast or to take to work for a snack.

Apple Cinnamon Cookie Teff Porridge

The word *teff* means "lost," because if you dropped a grain of teff, it is so small that it would be lost. This recipe calls for whole grain teff (not flour) and tastes like an apple cinnamon cookie. Yum!

Ingredients

½ cup whole grain teff

1½ cups filtered water

1 teaspoon coconut oil

⅛ teaspoon Himalayan salt

1–2 tablespoons chia seeds

1 organic apple, grated

Cinnamon to taste (I like to use a lot!)

¼ cup cashew milk or other alternative milk (for serving)

½ teaspoon raw local honey, coconut nectar, and/or a few drops of stevia liquid (for drizzling)

1 tablespoon raisins (optional)

1 tablespoon hemp hearts to top (optional)

Directions

1. Set a heavy, medium-sized saucepan over medium heat.

2. Put the teff into the saucepan and toast, stirring frequently until the grains begin to pop, about 3–6 minutes. (You will notice little white dots of popped grain but may not hear the popping, although you might begin to smell a mild toasty aroma.)

3. Meanwhile bring the water to a boil in a kettle or another saucepan.

4. Remove the teff from the heat, and stand back while you add the boiling water (because it can splatter). Also add the coconut oil and salt. Stir well. Put back onto the heat (medium low), cover, and cook at a medium-low simmer for 10 minutes. Stir from time to time to prevent the grains from sticking to the bottom. Mash any lumps against the side of the pan.

5. In the last minute of cooking, stir in the chia seeds and grated apple, and sprinkle on the cinnamon.

6. Add the milk alternative and drizzle of coconut nectar or other natural sweetener, top with hemp hearts and raisins (if using), and serve. (Remember, stevia can be bitter, so if you are using this as your sweetener, go easy.)

Make ahead tip: Make a double or triple batch so you have extra for the next day or so. This dish can be eaten cold or reheated.

Detox Drinks and Nondairy Milks

Herbal or Decaf Tea with Coconut Oil

Craving something sweet? Herbal tea with coconut oil is a great craving buster! It's not sweet itself, but I have found that it can get rid of a sugar craving. Brew your choice of herbal or decaf tea in water, and add 1–2 teaspoons of coconut oil. Allow to cool slightly before drinking to make sure the oil is not too hot. Don't like coconut oil? Replace it with almond, sesame, macadamia nut, or avocado oil.

Some yummy options:

- Decaf chai tea with coconut oil and coconut milk (a great replacement for the afternoon Starbucks run)

- Chamomile tea with coconut oil (a relaxing option for settling down in the evening)

Quick Pick-Me-Up Drink/Snack

Need a good on-the-go option? This is great for those days that are just jam-packed, or if you are traveling. Put 1 scoop of plant-based protein powder, ½–1 scoop greens powder (such as Green Vibrance), and 1–2 tablespoons chia seeds into a big glass jar or water bottle with at least 12 ounces water or a combination of water and coconut water. Shake well. Allow to soak for 5 minutes, and then enjoy. Optionally add a pinch of Himalayan salt. Sometimes, I will put all the dry ingredients into a baggie or container, and bring it with me to mix in case I need a quick pick-me-up on the go!

Artichoke Tea

Naturally detoxifying and supportive of the liver and digestive system, this tea can be served warm or cold.

Ingredients

1 organic artichoke

8–10 cups filtered water

Optional

1-inch piece gingerroot, peeled

1 small piece turmeric root, peeled

Juice from 1 lemon

Stevia or natural sweetener to taste (if desired)

Directions

1. Rinse the artichoke well, getting in between the leaves. Then cut into 4 sections lengthwise.

2. Put the artichoke pieces into a big pot of filtered water, and bring to a boil. (If you are using the ginger and turmeric, add those as well.)

3. Reduce to a low-medium simmer and cook for 20 minutes.

4. Take pot off the heat, and remove the artichoke.

5. Allow the liquid to cool slightly, about 20 minutes.

6. Run the tea through a strainer into a glass pitcher or jar to store in refrigerator. This tea should turn a beautiful deep green color. If it is brown, you might have cooked it too long, or at too high of a temperature. Make sure that the tea has cooled completely before storing.

If you cannot find organic artichokes, I suggest buying organic artichoke tea bags. Note that artichoke is a member of the thistle family, so if you are allergic to thistle, artichoke tea may not be for you. Also, artichoke tea can lower cholesterol, so those already on cholesterol-lowering medication (or with low cholesterol) should avoid artichoke tea.

Golden Milk Tea

This tea contains turmeric, which is a powerful anti-inflammatory spice that can support liver detoxification and assist in the removal of mucus. It is also a wonderful herbal remedy to treat stiff, sore, arthritic, or inflamed joints. Turmeric is a digestive tonic, antiseptic, antiparasitic, astringent, pain reliever, blood purifier, wound healer, kidney stone dissolver, eczema treatment, and more.

Ingredients

¼ teaspoon turmeric powder

¼ cup filtered water

1 cup cashew, almond, hemp, or coconut milk

Cinnamon, cardamom, ginger to taste (optional)

1 teaspoon coconut or almond oil (or more as desired)

Raw honey, coconut nectar, and/or stevia to taste

Directions

1. Place ¼ cup filtered water and turmeric powder in a small, heavy-bottom saucepan and bring to a boil, stirring for about 5–8 minutes until almost no liquid is left. Watch to make sure it does not burn!

2. Add the milk (and other spices) to the saucepan and heat until the milk just starts to comes to a boil. Then reduce heat and simmer for a few minutes.

3. Stir in the almond or coconut oil just after taking the pan off the heat. Start with 1 teaspoon; you may gradually add more if you like.

4. Add a small amount (¼–½ teaspoon) of raw honey or a few drops of stevia liquid.

5. Allow to cool just a bit, and serve. (Be careful because the oil can be very hot initially.)

As with all herbs and supplements, please consult your doctor if you are on medication before taking this tea. Herbs can be very powerful and may interfere and interact with medications. Turmeric can be a uterine stimulant, those who are pregnant should avoid it.

Bragg Lemonade

This beverage supports digestion and liver and gallbladder function.

Ingredients

1–2 teaspoons Bragg raw apple cider vinegar

Juice from ½ lemon

8 ounces water (ideally not too cold)

Pinch Himalayan salt

A couple drops of stevia or ¼ teaspoon raw honey or another natural sweetener to taste (optional)

Fresh Cashew Cream/Milk

(See below for a quick "cheater's" nut milk using cashew butter.)

Ingredients

1 cup raw unsalted organic cashews

4 cups water (Adjust amount of water depending on how thick you like it, you can always add more water, even before serving it.)

Himalayan salt (for soaking)

⅛ teaspoon vanilla extract (optional)

½ teaspoon coconut nectar or raw honey (or a few drops of stevia)

⅛–¼ teaspoon Himalayan salt

Optional

1–2 teaspoons white chia seeds (soak for 5 minutes)

1–2 teaspoons tahini (excellent calcium source)

Dash of cinnamon, nutmeg, or cardamom

Directions

1. Cover the cashews in 2 cups of water, sprinkle in a few shakes of Himalayan salt, and soak for 1–6 hours (no longer than 12 hours).

2. Drain and discard the soaking water.

3. Put 2 cups of filtered water, the soaked cashews, sweetener, salt, and optional ingredients into a blender and blend well to thoroughly combine and get rid of texture.

4. If desired, strain through a cheesecloth or chinois strainer, and chill.

5. Store in refrigerator in a glass jar or container for up to 3 days.

For quick nut milk, replace the raw cashews with 2–4 tablespoons of cashew or another nut butter. Proceed with steps 3–5.

See below for how to make cashew cheese.

Other Types of Nondairy Milk

Replace the cashews in the above recipe with:

- **Almond.** A harder nut than cashews, almonds should be soaked for 12–24 hours (changing water every 8–12 hours). If you want a whiter-colored milk, peel the dark skins off after soaking. After blending, strain through a cheesecloth or chinois strainer to collect the excess pulp. (I keep the pulp and add it to smoothies or season it and use it as a dip).

- **Coconut.** Soak ½ cup unsweetened dried coconut flesh in water for about 3 hours. You can also scoop out and blend raw coconut flesh.

- **Chia and hemp seeds.** Soak ¼ cup white chia seeds and ¼ cup hemp seeds for up to 3 hours.

Fresh-Pressed Juices

A quick way to boost your antioxidants and your alkalinity is to have a few fresh-pressed juices during phase two! Drinking these on an empty stomach is good—or even better, take with a source of healthy fat to aid in the absorption of the fat-soluble vitamins and keep the blood sugar level. Stir in 2 tablespoons of chia seeds, a teaspoon of avocado oil, or eat with a handful of nuts. Because each 8-ounce glass can contain between 2–3 pounds of produce, it is important to use only *organic* vegetables and fruits for fresh juices.

Some Juicing Recipe Ideas

- **Detoxing Green Lemonade:** 1 green apple, 1 small slice peeled ginger, 1 lemon (most of peel removed), 5–6 kale leaves (or kale and spinach), 1 small cucumber, 1–2 celery stalks, handful of parsley

- **Rainbow Veggie Blend:** 1 carrot, 1 small raw beet, 1 green apple, 1–2 stalks celery, handful of leafy greens (such as romaine, kale, spinach)

- **Tropical Green Drink:** 1 medium cucumber, 1 celery stalk, handful of kale or leafy greens, 1 peeled lime, ¼ cup chopped pineapple, handful of parsley

Directions

1. Pass the vegetables and fruits through a juicer. If you don't have one, you can use a blender and just pour the blend through a fine strainer.

2. Drink right away, and store any extra in the refrigerator for up to 1 day.

    Note: If you drink beet juice or eat a lot of beets, it is totally normal to see a bright beet color in the toilet when you have a bowel movement. Do not worry: it is not blood; it is the beets. This can actually help you to determine the "transit time" of your foods, which is an indicator of how long they are taking to get through the colon. An ideal transit time is about 12–24 hours. Longer, and your body could be holding on to toxins. Less, and you might not be absorbing nutrients. Beets are excellent for supporting the liver.

Dips, Dressings, and Crackers

Garlic Herbed Cashew Cheese

This is a soft spreadable and dippable nondairy "cheese" dip.

Ingredients

1 cup raw cashews (not salted or roasted)

2 teaspoons raw cider vinegar

2½ cups filtered water

1 teaspoon lemon juice

⅛ teaspoon sea salt (or more as preferred)

2–3 cloves garlic

Dill, basil, or other herbs to taste

Paprika or your favorite spice to taste

1 teaspoon nutritional yeast (optional; often in health food supplement sections—do not use active or brewer's yeast!)

Directions

1. Soak cashews in 2 cups of water for at least 3 hours or overnight.

2. Drain off the liquid.

3. Put cashews into a blender, add ½ cup of water, vinegar, lemon juice, salt, garlic, desired herbs and spices, and nutritional yeast (if using).

4. Blend well until incorporated with a smooth texture.

   Chipotle variation: Use 1 clove garlic, no herbs, and add in 1 teaspoon of chipotle powder.

   Store in an airtight container in the refrigerator for up to 3 days. Some separation can occur after storing, so just stir before serving.

Quick Artichoke Pesto Dip

Ingredients

12 oz. bag (about 2 ½ cups) frozen artichoke hearts, thawed (available at Trader Joe's)

½ cup pine nuts (toasted in 350-degree oven for approx. 15 minutes)—walnuts work well too

3–4 cloves garlic

3–4 tablespoons fresh lemon juice

2–3 tablespoons extra virgin olive oil

2 cups loosely packed basil leaves

1 teaspoon sea salt

Paprika to taste (optional)

Directions

Put all ingredients into a food processor and blend together to create a paste. Taste and adjust for seasoning/salt. More olive oil will make it creamier. Great cold as a dip for veggies or chia crackers. Can also be baked in a 350-degree oven for 15 minutes to create a hot dip. Or spread it on top of cooked chicken or fish.

Hummus Dip

Ingredients

1 can (16 ounces, about 1½ cups) garbanzo beans

2 cloves garlic

¼ cup fresh squeezed lemon juice

1 tablespoon tahini (sesame paste)

¾ teaspoon sea salt

¼ teaspoon fresh cracked pepper

¼ cup olive oil

Directions

1. Put everything except the olive oil into a food processor and process until well combined. Then add olive oil slowly to create a paste.

2. Taste and adjust for seasoning/salt. More olive oil will make it creamier.

Optional: Make a red pepper hummus, by adding some roasted red peppers. Or add black or green olives for an olive hummus.

For the garbanzo beans (chickpeas): Sometimes you can find them in a box, which I prefer using over canned. Or you can soak and cook them yourself from dried.

Chia and Pumpkin Seed Crackers

Ingredients

½ cup cashew or blanched almond meal/flour

⅓ cup chia seeds (can use ground or whole)

⅓ cup pumpkin seeds (or another nut/seed), chopped

½ teaspoon good-quality salt (divided)

¼ cup water

2 teaspoons coconut oil (melted to liquid)

Herbs/spices of your choice (rosemary or paprika work)

Directions

1. Preheat the oven to 350 degrees, and line a baking sheet with parchment paper.

2. Mix together the nut flour, chia seeds, chopped pumpkin seeds, ¼ teaspoon of the salt, water, and coconut oil in a bowl. Let it rest for about 5 minutes.

3. Scoop out teaspoonfuls, and using oiled hands, roll into balls and press down to flatten them onto the parchment sheet to make them as thin as you can. Once they are all on the pan, sprinkle on remaining ¼ teaspoon salt and any spices and/or herbs you choose.

4. Put into middle-upper section of oven for about 20 minutes. Flip them over and cook another 8–10 minutes or until just lightly browning on the edges and crispy.

5. Store extras in an airtight container.

Quick (Vinegar-Free) Lemon Herb Vinaigrette or Marinade

This is great on salads, as a marinade, or to pour over baked or grilled chicken or fish just before serving.

Ingredients

1 clove garlic, finely minced, or 1 teaspoon minced shallots

½ cup fresh lemon juice (juice from approx. 1 large lemon)

¼ cup chopped fresh herbs (such as oregano and basil, or rosemary for a marinade)

Salt and pepper to taste

⅓ cup olive or avocado oil

½ teaspoon raw honey (or a few drops stevia or combination of the two)

Directions

Whisk together all the ingredients except the olive oil in a blender or bowl, or shake up in a jar. Continue to whisk and slowly add the olive oil. This will emulsify and thicken the dressing to keep it from separating. Taste and adjust salt and pepper.

Green Goddess Dressing

Ingredients

1 clove garlic

2 tablespoons raw Bragg apple cider vinegar

1 tablespoon Dijon mustard

2 tablespoons walnuts, almonds, pumpkin seeds, or pine nuts

2 teaspoons raw honey or coconut palm nectar, or a few drops stevia

3 teaspoons fresh lemon juice

½ teaspoon sea salt

Ground black pepper to taste

¼ cup fresh dill, basil, and/or arugula

½ cup extra virgin olive oil or avocado oil

Directions

1. Put garlic, vinegar, mustard, pine nuts, honey, salt and pepper into blender and blend to combine well.

2. Add in dill or other green herb and then drizzle in olive oil slowly while blending to emulsify. (This is the secret to using olive oil—if you emulsify it, it will not separate.)

3. Put into a bottle and chill in refrigerator.

4. Pull out about 10 minutes before using to loosen up the dressing, and shake well.

Quick Lemony Walnut Pesto

Saves in the refrigerator for up to 3 days. It can also be frozen.

Ingredients

1 cup parsley

1 cup basil

1–2 cloves garlic

½ cup raw walnuts, toasted in 350-degree oven till lightly browned

Zest of 1 lemon (organic)

2 tablespoons lemon juice

5–6 tablespoons olive oil

Directions

Pulse all the ingredients except olive oil in a food processor until finely chopped. Then slowly add in the olive oil and process until combined.

Balsamic Dressing

Ingredients

1 tablespoon Dijon mustard

1 tablespoon Bragg raw apple cider vinegar

3 tablespoons balsamic vinegar

½ teaspoon sea salt

Fresh or dried herbs such as parsley, oregano, etc.

Ground black pepper to taste

½ cup extra virgin olive oil or avocado oil

Directions

1. Put all the ingredients except the oil into a blender, and blend to combine well.
2. Drizzle in olive oil slowly while blending to emulsify.
3. Put into a bottle and chill in the refrigerator.
4. Pull out about 10 minutes before using to loosen up the dressing, and shake well.

"Cheesy" Kale Chips

Ingredients

1 head organic curly kale

Olive oil to taste

Sea or Himalayan salt and pepper

Dried herbs of your choice

Nutritional yeast to taste (approximately 2 tablespoons)

Directions

1. Preheat the oven to 350 degrees.

2. Break apart the kale leaves into bite-sized pieces. Remove and discard the stems and hard spines.

3. Drizzle olive oil onto the kale and sprinkle with sea salt and fresh cracked pepper.

4. Massage the kale to make sure each piece is lightly coated with oil and salt/pepper.

5. Optionally, sprinkle on garlic, other herbs, and nutritional yeast as well.

6. Put kale on a baking sheet and bake on the middle rack approx. 10–15 minutes. Should still be slightly green, but crispy. Be careful to not burn.

Soups, Salads, and Lunch

Soups are wonderfully healing, warming, alkalizing, hydrating, and comforting. Make the broth on the weekend, and you have lunch for several days.

Organic Slow-Cooked Chicken Bone Broth

An essential when someone has a cold, organic bone broth is also very healing to the gut and immune system. The longer a bone broth cooks, the more collagen is released from the bones, and the more healing it is to the gut. I like to turn this broth into a Mexican soup and add avocado to boost the fat and keep me satisfied longer. See below for that option!

Ingredients

2 bone-in *organic* chicken breasts and/or 3–4 bone-in thighs (You can also throw in some more bones—neck, feet, etc.—the more bones, the better/tastier.)

1 tablespoon Celtic salt, or Himalayan salt

1 onion, cut into quarters

3–4 carrots

3–4 celery stalks

2 bay leaves

1 tablespoon Bragg raw apple cider vinegar (pulls collagen and nutrients from bones)

3–4 thyme sprigs

14 cups water (or as much as your pot can hold!)

Big handful of parsley

1 kombu strip (optional; found in natural foods stores near seaweed, adds a rich "umami" taste and boosts natural minerals and iodine to support thyroid function and digestion.)

Directions

1. Season the chicken lightly with 1 teaspoon of high-quality sea salt.

2. Cut the onion, carrots, and celery into large chunks.

3. Put all of the following in a heavy pot on the stove: the onion, carrot, celery, vinegar, thyme sprigs, salt, chicken (with extra bones if using), and kombu strip (if using). Cover with the filtered water.

4. On high heat, bring to a boil. Then change to low heat and simmer partially covered with a lid for about 2 hours (or until the chicken is cooked through, depending on how large your chicken pieces are).

5. Take out the chicken and cut into it to see if it is cooked through. If it is not, return it to the pot to cook for another 20 minutes.

6. When the chicken is done and cool enough to touch, remove the meat, and shred or chop it. Store it in the refrigerator for use in soup, salads, etc.

7. Strain out the onion, kombu, celery, and carrots (and bones if not cooking them longer).

8. Skim off any foam from the top of the pot. *If you want to use the broth at this point, skip to step 10. Otherwise, cooking the bones longer will extract more minerals and collagen.*

9. Return the broth and chicken bones to the pot or a slow cooker, and cook on simmer or low for another 3–12 hours. Skim off any foam from the top.

10. Taste the broth, and add salt if needed. (If it is too salty, just add a little more water.)

11. Store the broth in glass containers in the refrigerator for up to 4 days or in the freezer for up to 3 months.

Mexican Chicken Soup

Put the chicken broth from the previous recipe into a pot, bring to a simmer, and add the following.

Ingredients

½ cup shredded chicken (from making broth)

4–5 chopped grape tomatoes

Big handful baby spinach, chopped

Chopped organic cilantro to taste

Fresh jalapeño, minced, to taste (optional)

Ancho chili or smoked paprika powder (a couple shakes or to taste)

Pour into a bowl and add before serving:

Fresh avocado, cut into chunks and scooped out

Juice from a wedge of a lime

Detoxifying Veggie Soup

This soup is quick and easy to make and contains turmeric, which is an incredibly powerful anti-inflammatory and antioxidant herb. Fresh dill (one of the garnishes used here) has been shown to be helpful for relieving headaches, so it is the perfect addition for those trying to wean off of caffeine, which can cause headaches.

If you need soup broth for a recipe, simply strain out the vegetables and store the extra in an airtight container in the refrigerator.

Ingredients

1 onion chopped

3 tablespoons coconut or olive oil

1 cup diced celery

1 cup diced carrots

1 tablespoon sea or Himalayan salt

1 teaspoon turmeric powder

1 bay leaf

10 cups filtered water

1 cup diced zucchini

Directions

1. In a large heavy-bottom saucepan, sauté the onion in the oil on low heat until tender, about 5 minutes.
2. Add in the celery, carrots, salt, turmeric, bay leaf, and 10 cups of filtered water.
3. Bring to a boil, then reduce to a simmer and cook approximately 20 minutes.
4. Add in the zucchini and simmer 5 minutes more.
5. Remove bay leaf before serving/storing.
6. When ready to serve, you can add the following garnishes to the hot soup.

Garnishes (Per Serving)

Add the following to approximately 1 cup of broth:

½ cup baby spinach or other dark leafy green, chopped

3 tablespoons chopped fresh dill

1 tablespoon fresh lemon juice

½ avocado, lightly salted with sea salt

Put the spinach and dill in a large bowl, and pour the steaming hot broth over the garnishes. Cover the bowl and let steam for about 3-4 minutes. Then add the squeeze of fresh lemon and avocado chunks right before serving.

Note: My kids like this yummy veggie broth over some cooked brown rice pasta. Add some shredded cooked chicken, and you have a quick homemade chicken soup.

Power Greens Soup

Serves 2 as a side dish, or 1 for a main course.

This detoxifying soup is **the bomb!** It is super quick and easy to make—coming together in 10 minutes.

Ingredients

1-2 tablespoons olive, avocado, or coconut oil

1 garlic clove, chopped

3 cups "power greens" (mixed leafy greens of kale, spinach, chard, etc.)

Juice from ⅓ lemon (or lime)

Good-quality salt

1 cup broth (you could use your homemade broth or a low-sodium store-bought vegetable or free-range chicken stock)

½ organic cucumber or 1 small organic pickling cucumber

1 stalk celery

Small bunch of parsley (optional)

2 tablespoons chia seeds

Coconut milk/cream or cashew cream for serving

Aleppo peppers or cayenne (to taste)

Directions

1. Heat a pan on medium, put in oil, and then add in garlic. Sauté for about 2 minutes, and then add in greens. Squeeze on the lemon juice and salt to taste. Sauté until greens are just wilted.

2. Put everything from the pan into the blender, add in the broth (can warm up on stovetop ahead of time), raw cucumber, celery stalk, and parsley if using. Blend on high for a few minutes until soup is steaming.

3. Pour the soup into bowl(s). Swirl 1–2 tablespoons of coconut milk or coconut cream into center of bowl. Top with aleppo peppers, cayenne, or fresh cracked black pepper to taste. Serve!

Dandelion and Beet Detox Salad

Serves 2-4 people.

Beets, dandelion greens, and pumpkin seeds all support the body to detoxify. This is delicious with the Green Goddess Dressing!

Ingredients

3 small beets, roasted in 400-degree oven until tender

1½ cups mixed greens or baby spinach

1½ cups dandelion greens

1 firm-ripe avocado, salted and cut into chunks

¼ cup pepitas (pumpkin seeds)

¼ cup grated carrots

Directions

1. Roast the beets in a 400-degree oven ahead of time; the skins should peel off easily. Slice or dice them when ready to serve (can be served cold or warm). Do this step ahead of time so they are ready when you need them; they store in the refrigerator for up to 3 days.

2. Rinse and chop all the greens and transfer to a large salad bowl. Add avocado, pumpkin seeds, and grated carrots.

3. Drizzle vinaigrette or Green Goddess Dressing over greens and beets, and toss to combine.

Everything but the Kitchen Sink Salad

This is the salad for using up leftovers. Just throw in whatever veggies, quinoa, and/or chicken you have in the fridge! Roasted broccoli, sautéed beans, grilled zucchini—just go for it! If you don't have leftovers, chop up whatever veggies you like, such as red pepper, cucumber, etc.

Ingredients

2 cups mixed greens or baby spinach

Leftover roasted veggies, chopped

Leftover quinoa

Leftover chicken or another protein

Handful pumpkin seeds, pine nuts, or other chopped nut (optional)

½ firm-ripe avocado, lightly salted and cut into chunks

Finely chopped or grated carrots

Diced red pepper

Diced cucumbers

Fresh pepper to taste

Directions

1. Rinse and chop the greens, and transfer to a large salad bowl. Add in whatever leftovers you are using—veggies, quinoa, chicken.

2. Drizzle some vinaigrette over the salad and toss to combine. Sprinkle with nuts, avocado chunks, carrots, peppers, cucumber, and fresh cracked pepper, and serve immediately.

Chicken Salad in Lettuce Cups

Ingredients

Cooked chicken, chopped or shredded (A great way to use leftovers from your soup broth! *You can also swap chicken for tuna if you look for lower mercury varieties like skipjack or Wild Planet brand tuna.*)

2–3 tablespoons soy-free Vegenaise mayonnaise

Fresh lemon juice to taste

1 teaspoon Dijon mustard

¼ cup finely chopped celery

¼ cup chopped apples

¼ cup almond slivers (optional; roast in a 350-degree oven first)

Fresh cracked pepper to taste

Chopped or dried parsley to taste

Butter lettuce leaves or Swiss chard

Directions

1. Prep and mix all the ingredients except the lettuce.

2. Put mixture into the lettuce cups, or wrap into chard.

3. Serve and enjoy!

    Make ahead tips: Make a double or triple recipe of the chicken salad, and you will have some for another lunch this week! Add it to one of your salads!

Side Dishes

You might notice that there are a lot of recipes for side dishes and veggies. During the Perfect Metabolism Plan, you should increase your intake of plant-based foods. So go ahead and make the veggies the star of your plate! Emphasizing plant-based foods helps you to alkalize your body, improve digestion, and boost your intake of antioxidants, vitamins, and minerals.

Cauliflower Rice

Using cauliflower rice is an easy way to cut down on your grains, but keep the "feel" of them! Wonderful with curry and stir-fries and as a side dish.

Ingredients

1 head organic cauliflower

2–3 tablespoons coconut oil and/or grass-fed ghee

Salt and pepper to taste

Directions

1. Roughly cut the cauliflower into florets and put them into the food processor.

2. Pulse until they are finely chopped and resemble rice grains.

3. Heat up a large skillet (a heavy cast-iron skillet works best), and melt the coconut oil and/or ghee over medium heat.

4. Add in the cauliflower "rice" and cook for about 5 minutes. Then sprinkle with salt and pepper. *(Add other spices if desired.)*

5. Cook until it is just starting to turn light golden brown and is tender but not too mushy.

6. Add more salt and pepper to taste, and any other seasonings that you like.

Options

Finely mince an onion and sauté for 5 minutes before adding in the cauliflower rice.

Make coconut lime "rice" by adding in ¼ cup toasted unsweetened coconut flakes, 2 tablespoons lime juice, and 2 tablespoons coconut milk in the last few minutes of cooking. Add in some chopped cilantro if desired.

Baked Mashed Cauliflower "Potatoes"

Ingredients

1 head cauliflower, cut into florets

2 tablespoons your choice nondairy milk (unsweetened)

2 tablespoons olive oil (I love using infused oils for this to give it more flavor) or melted coconut oil

2 tablespoons nutritional yeast (optional; gives a nice nutty cheesy flavor, boosts B vitamins)

Salt and pepper to taste

1 clove garlic (optional; roast in oven ahead of time if desired)

Directions

1. Steam the cauliflower in a steaming pot over simmering water on the stovetop until fork-tender, about 7 minutes. (It should be mashable, but not mushy.)

2. Put into a food processor or use a hand mixer, and gradually add the nondairy milk, olive oil, nutritional yeast, and salt and some. If using, add in the raw or roasted garlic.

3. Mix it all together until you have achieved the desired texture.

4. Taste. Add more seasoning if needed. (Do not be afraid to add salt to please your taste buds—as long as it is high-quality salt.)

5. Serve immediately. Or if you are making the baked version, spread into an eight-by-eight baking dish that has been lightly greased with olive or coconut oil. Bake in a 425-degree oven for 20 minutes or until the edges are slightly browning.

Lemony Green Beans

This is a favorite go-to veggie side dish. It works with everything!

Ingredients

1 pound fresh green beans, ends snipped

1–2 tablespoons ghee or olive or coconut oil (or a combination)

1 shallot, minced (optional)

Fresh lemon juice (to taste)

Sea salt and pepper (gray sea salt is amazing on this recipe)

Directions

1. Put the green beans into a sauté pan with about 1 inch of water on the bottom.

2. Cover with a lid, bring to a boil, and steam for about 3–5 minutes, or until they are bright green and just fork-tender.

3. Drain out the water, add the ghee or coconut oil and shallots (if using), and sauté for a few minutes until the shallots are cooked and the green beans are tender but not mushy.

4. Squeeze on the lemon juice, and season to taste with salt and fresh cracked pepper. Enjoy!

Ratatouille

Ingredients

1 yellow, white, or sweet onion

2–3 tablespoons coconut oil, ghee, or avocado oil (or a combination)

1–2 cloves garlic, chopped or pressed (optional)

1 container button mushrooms, sliced or chopped

1 red pepper, chopped

3 cups baby spinach leaves, chopped

Salt and pepper to taste

Directions

1. Slice the onion in half, and then slice the halves into thin half moons.

2. Heat a pan over medium heat and add the oil.

3. Sauté the onion for about 7 minutes until it just starts to caramelize a bit. Then add the garlic and mushrooms, and cook those for about 2–3 minutes.

4. Add the red pepper, and cook for a couple minutes more.

5. Add the spinach in the last 1–2 minutes of cooking, until just wilted. Salt and pepper to taste.

Garlic Sautéed Power Greens

Serves 3-4

Ingredients

2 tablespoons coconut oil

2–3 cloves garlic, chopped

4 cups chopped "power greens" (kale, spinach, chard, etc.)

Juice from ½ a lemon

Sea or Himalayan salt

Fresh cracked pepper

Trader Joe's 21 Seasoning blend

Aleppo pepper to taste (optional)

Directions

1. Heat a pan on medium, and put in the coconut oil.
2. Put the garlic in the pan and sauté for a minute; then add the greens.
3. Squeeze on lemon juice, add in the salt and pepper to taste, and any other seasoning you choose.
4. Cook until greens are wilted.

Sweet Potato Wedges

Ingredients

3 large organic sweet potatoes

2 tablespoons avocado or melted coconut oil

Sea salt and cracked pepper

Smoked paprika (or aleppo pepper if you can find it) (optional)

Directions

1. Preheat the oven to 425 degrees.
2. Rinse the potatoes and scrub off any dirt.
3. Cut into 1-inch wedges, and dry the wedges really well with a paper towel.
4. Toss the potato wedges in the oil, and season with salt, pepper, and smoked paprika.
5. Roast on a large cookie sheet for 20–25 minutes, turning once or twice.

Roasted Broccoli and Cauliflower

Ingredients

2–3 heads broccoli (plus 1 small head cauliflower), cut into pieces

Olive or avocado oil

Sea or Himalayan salt and fresh cracked pepper

Paprika, cayenne or aleppo pepper if you like a little spice (optional)

Directions

1. Preheat the oven to 400 degrees.

2. Coat the vegetables well with oil, and season well with salt and pepper. Sprinkle on paprika, cayenne, or aleppo pepper if using.

3. Roast for about 20 minutes or until fork-tender, turning once halfway through.

Dinners/Main Courses

Pesto Paleo Pasta

Serves 2.

This is one of my weeknight staples. I love my spiral slicer for making zucchini noodles!

Ingredients

4 small organic zucchini (or alternatively 1 spaghetti squash)

Quick Lemony Walnut Pesto or Quick Artichoke Pesto Dip

Directions

Cut the zucchini into "spaghetti noodles" using a spiral slicer. You can also use a mandoline or a vegetable peeler and make wider "noodles." These can be served raw with walnut or artichoke pesto stirred in. (My kids lick the plate with this recipe!) Or you can drop them into boiling water for about 3–5 minutes, and drain well. (I use a paper towel to squeeze out the water)

Spaghetti squash version: Pierce the squash with a knife a few times, and put it into a preheated 400-degree oven. Cook for about 50 minutes to 1 hour, or until fork-tender. (*Note:* It cooks faster if you cut it in half first, and place it flesh side down on the pan.) Remove it from oven and allow to cool for 10 minutes. Cut the squash open and remove the seeds and pulp. Shred the squash with a fork into "noodles."

Top your zucchini or spaghetti squash Paleo noodles with your choice of pesto (see recipes). Alternatively, you could use a high-quality marinara sauce (after checking the label to make sure it does not have added sugar or soy oil).

Wild Salmon with Mustard and Dill Sauce

Serves 4

This is one of our family's staple recipes. It is easy to make and pleases everyone!

Serve it with Cauliflower Rice or quinoa and Lemony Green Beans, or grilled zucchini with dill!

Ingredients

1 ½-pound wild salmon filet (Or if you choose farmed, make sure it is from a reputable grocery store that does not add artificial colorings or use synthetics in the feed.)

Avocado oil (to lightly coat the fish)

Salt and pepper

Fresh (or dried) dill

Mustard and Dill Sauce

4 tablespoons Dijon mustard

1 tablespoon Bragg raw apple cider vinegar

Juice from one lemon (about 3 tablespoons)

1–2 teaspoons raw honey or coconut palm nectar, or a few drops stevia (or a combo)

¼ teaspoon sea salt and fresh cracked pepper to taste

⅓ cup virgin cold-pressed olive oil

¼ cup fresh dill

Directions

1. Preheat the grill (or the oven to 400 degrees).

2. Lightly coat the fish with the oil, and then season it with sea salt, pepper, and chopped dill.

3. For the dressing, put the all the ingredients except the olive oil and dill into a blender or food processor, and blend to combine.

4. Bake the fish in the top quarter of the oven at 400 degrees for approx. 10 minutes. Or grill it approx. 4–5 minutes a side on a medium high heat.

5. Slowly drizzle in the olive oil, continuing to blend to emulsify. Once the sauce has thickened, add in the dill and blend to just chop the dill. Do not blend too long, or the sauce will turn green (although it still tastes good that way!).

Pesto Fish Baked in Parchment

Excellent served with quinoa or Cauliflower Rice and a salad of your choice.

Ingredients

2 filets wild halibut or another white fish

Olive or avocado oil

Sea salt and fresh pepper or thinly sliced red Thai chilis

4 tablespoons artichoke or walnut pesto (see pesto recipe)

2 zucchini, grated

2 carrots, grated

2 tablespoons fresh lemon juice

Directions

1. Preheat the oven to 425 degrees.

2. Lightly brush the oil on the fish and season with salt and pepper.

3. Place each fillet on a piece of parchment paper (you can also do this in an ovenproof baking dish if you prefer), and spread 2 tablespoons of the pesto on each filet.
4. Top each filet with grated zucchini and carrots.
5. Drizzle with some lemon juice, then seal up the parchment into little "packages." You can even staple them to close. Bake for approximately 12–15 minutes.

Other options for topping the fish
Italian style: Capers, chopped olives, lemon, and fresh thyme
Asian style: Fresh grated ginger, tamari, sesame oil with grated carrot and cabbage

Balsamic Chicken

Serves 2.
This dish is wonderful served with Cauliflower Rice or quinoa, and it's also great leftover in a salad—so make extra!

Ingredients

2 boneless, skinless chicken breasts, or thighs if you prefer

Salt and pepper to taste

2 tablespoons avocado oil, ghee, or coconut oil

2 tablespoons chopped garlic

¼ cup balsamic vinegar

1 cup organic grape tomatoes

¼ cup chopped fresh basil

Directions

1. Season the chicken breasts with salt and pepper.
2. Put 2 tablespoons of oil or ghee (or combination) in a preheated pan.
3. Sauté the chicken for about 5 minutes a side on medium high. It should be lightly browned and cooked through.

4. Remove the chicken from the pan, set on a plate, and cover with foil to keep warm.

5. Sauté the chopped garlic in the pan for about 1 minute (add a little more oil first if needed). Take off the heat for a second, very carefully add in the balsamic vinegar (it can spatter), and then add in the grape/cherry tomatoes and return the pan to the stovetop over a low-medium heat.

6. Sauté until the tomatoes start to get soft and the balsamic vinegar reduces just a little.

7. Add in the fresh basil and just stir around a couple times.

8. Serve the chicken with the sauce and tomatoes.

Zucchini Pizza Crust

This works best on a pizza stone. *Also note:* This recipe uses eggs.

Ingredients

2 organic or pastured eggs

2 tablespoons chia seeds (I like to use ground chia seeds for this, ground flax also works.)

2 small zucchini (organic)

½ cup garbanzo bean (chickpea) flour

1 tablespoon coconut oil, melted (You will need a little more for the pizza stone)

½ teaspoon good-quality salt

Fresh cracked pepper to taste

1 garlic clove, pressed, or garlic powder

½ teaspoon dried Italian herbs such as basil and oregano

Directions

1. Put your pizza stone or pan into the oven, and preheat the oven to 425 degrees.

2. Crack the eggs into a bowl and whisk them. Add in the chia seeds and let soak for a few minutes.

3. Now grate the zucchini.

4. Add the zucchini and the rest of the ingredients to the eggs, and stir to combine.

5. Take the preheated pizza stone out of the oven. Coat the cooking area with coconut oil. Spoon the dough evenly onto the stone.

6. Put the pizza stone into the lower third of the oven to bake for about 8 minutes.

7. Move it up to the bottom of the upper third of the oven (not too close to the top). Cook for another 5–8 minutes.

8. After this it should be fairly firm and cooked through. If you put a spatula under it, it should not be soggy or bend too much.

9. Now it is ready to add your toppings. My favorite toppings are green olives, arugula, sautéed mushrooms, and onions. Lightly drizzle the with a little olive oil (about ½ teaspoon or so), or spread some pesto or a little marinara. You can add some sheep or goat cheese (if you are not off dairy).

10. Put the topped pizza into the oven and bake for about 8–10 minutes or until crust is lightly browned on the sides and the arugula or spinach is wilted—or if using cheese, it is melted.

    Optional: Drizzle with a little aged balsamic vinegar before serving.

    Make ahead idea: Make and bake the dough in advance, and store in the refrigerator till it is time to add the toppings.

Steak with Chimichurri Sauce

Serves 4.

This marinade is full of detoxifying parsley and garlic. Marinating meat before cooking it not only gives it a lot of flavor, but it also helps to prevent oxidation and free radical formation. (This sauce is also great on chicken or grilled fish.)

Ingredients

1 grass-fed organic flank or skirt steak (about 1½ pounds)

Chimichurri

1 cup organic parsley

6 cloves garlic

1 tablespoon fresh oregano

2 tablespoons fresh lemon juice

2 tablespoons of Bragg apple cider vinegar

3 tablespoons water

½ cup olive or avocado oil

Fresh cracked pepper and salt

Crushed aleppo peppers or red pepper flakes to taste

Directions

1. Put everything for the chimichurri into a food processor and blend together. This can be done ahead of time. Taste and adjust for spice and seasoning.

2. Spoon out a couple tablespoons of the chimichurri on the steak (or whatever protein you are using, such as chicken or fish) to marinate it for 10 minutes up to 4 hours for steak or chicken. Reserve the rest of the sauce for serving.

3. Grill the steak on medium-heat until done to your liking. Serve with more chimichurri sauce and whatever vegetable you like alongside. This goes great with grilled veggies like zucchini.

Desserts and Chocolates

Dark chocolate is a superfood, so it is allowed on the Perfect Metabolism program! But if you purchase it, make sure that you choose only 70 percent or higher cacao content. (And check that label for sugar and try to limit your intake to no more than 5 grams of sugar from dark chocolate daily.) Raw cacao chocolates are even better. There are also some stevia-sweetened brands. Or try these homemade chocolates or chocolate mousse, made with raw cacao and coconut oil.

Coconut Cacao Chocolates

These are not only delicious, but they also have an appetite-suppressing quality because of the healthy coconut oil! So make a batch, and when you are craving sweets, give one or two of these a try. You may notice you feel less hungry and more satisfied afterward. If you choose to add the maca powder, you will be supporting hormones and vitality through this adaptogen.

Equipment

Silicon mini ice cube tray or parchment-lined pan

Ingredients

⅔ cup virgin unrefined coconut oil

½ cup raw cacao powder *(Note: raw cacao is different from cocoa)*

24 drops stevia liquid

2 teaspoons of raw honey or coconut palm nectar

1 teaspoon pure vanilla extract

¼ teaspoon salt

2 teaspoons maca powder (optional; I use gelatinized, as it is better absorbed.)

2 tablespoons of almond butter (optional; add if you want a nutty chocolate, or you can add 1 teaspoon cinnamon for a Mexican-style chocolate)

Directions

1. In a small saucepan, melt the coconut oil over a very low heat. Remove from heat when it becomes liquid. Do not let it heat up too fast or on higher than a low setting. If it smokes, your heat is too high!

2. Mix all ingredients together to combine well (can be done in a blender).

3. Pour into molds or onto a parchment-lined pan.

4. Put them into the freezer for 10 minutes to solidify.

They are ready to eat—enjoy! I like to store these in the freezer (because coconut oil melts at 76 degrees, they need to be kept cold). If you want them to be stable at room temperature, substitute cocoa butter for the coconut oil.

Visit *www.perfectmetabolism.com* for a delicious recipe for Cacao Almond Butter Cups.

For those who cannot handle chocolate, replace the cacao with almond butter.

Cacao Mousse

Ingredients

½ cup coconut milk (or cashew or almond milk)

2 tablespoons chia seeds (soak in milk for 3–5 minutes)

½ firm, ripe avocado

1 teaspoon coconut oil

10 drops stevia (or combination of ½ teaspoon coconut nectar and stevia)

2–3 tablespoons raw cacao powder (to taste)

½ teaspoon vanilla extract, powder, or seeds from inside a vanilla bean pod

Small pinch Himalayan salt

Ice (optional)

Optional toppings:

Shredded unsweetened coconut

Chopped walnuts

Raw cacao nibs (taste like nutty chocolate chips)

Directions

Put all of the ingredients into a blender and blend until smooth. If serving right away, add a couple ice cubes to chill and make desired thickness, and blend again until smooth.

If you cannot handle or do not like chocolate, simply replace the cacao powder with lucuma powder for more of a caramel vanilla-flavored mousse. Because lucuma powder is sweet, you might want to adjust the honey or stevia proportions.

Sara's Cacao Snowballs

Ingredients

1 cup raw almonds (or another nut)

3-4 pitted dates, soaked in water for 5 minutes

¼ cup raw cacao powder

2 tablespoons chia seeds (soaked in ¼ cup water to make a gel)

¼ teaspoon Himalayan salt

½ cup shredded unsweetened coconut, plus more for rolling

1 tsp. vanilla extract or powder

1 tsp cinnamon

1 tablespoons coconut oil, melted

Optional

1 scoop greens powder

1 scoop vanilla protein powder

10 drops of stevia liquid, or 1 teaspoon of raw honey

Directions

1. If you have the time, soak the almonds in water for 6–12 hours. Drain the water and place the almonds on a paper towel and dry slightly.

2. Put the almonds in the food processor and process until very finely chopped.

4. Add the cacao, chia seeds, salt, and coconut, and pulse till mixed well. Add the optional ingredients

5. Add the coconut oil, chia gel, and the drained/soaked dates. Turn on the processor, the mixture should come together into a big lump. If it does not, add a little water.

6. Taste and adjust.

7. Roll into balls, and then roll the balls in the dried shredded coconut.

8. Store in an airtight container in the freezer for up to month, or refrigerator for up to 1 week.

Visit *www.perfectmetabolism.com* for more recipes, shopping lists, meal plans, and some recommended products/brands.

✒ Appendix ✒

Perfect Metabolism
Meal Plan Blank Form

DAY: _____			
Breakfast	*Lunch*	*Snack*	*Dinner*

Record how you are doing, thoughts, feelings, and cravings:

Evening Prep

| DAY: _____ |
Breakfast	Lunch	Snack	Dinner

Record how you are doing, thoughts, feelings, and cravings:

Evening Prep

✄ Resources ✁

Helpful Websites

www.chriskresser.com

www.ewg.org

www.foodbabe.com

www.mercola.com

www.nongmoproject.org

www.precisionnutrition.com

www.righttoknow-gmo.org

www.undergroundwellness.com

www.westonaprice.org

www.whfoods.com

Films/Documentaries

Fat, Sick and Nearly Dead

Fed Up

Food, Inc.

Food Matters

Genetic Roulette

GMO OMG

Hungry for Change

Stress: Portrait of a Killer

Recommended Reading

There are numerous books written entirely about each one of the keys in this book. If you are interested in delving more deeply into any of these topics—or other areas of health and nutrition—the following are highly recommended.

An A-Z Guide to Food Additives, Never Eat What You Can't Pronounce by Deanna Minich, PdD, CN

The Blood Sugar Solution (and several other books) by Dr. Mark Hyman

Clean (and Clean Gut) by Alejandro Junger, MD

Coconut Cures by Bruce Fife, ND

Dangerous Grains by James Braly, MD, and Ron Hoggan, MA

The Diet Cure by Julia Ross, MA

Eat Fat, Lose Fat by Dr. Mary Enig and Sally Fallon

The Fast Diet by Dr. Michael Mosley

Food Matters by Mark Bittman

Food Rules by Michael Pollan

Grain Brain by Dr. David Perlmutter

The Great Cholesterol Myth by Dr. Stephen Sinatra and Jonny Bowden, PhD

The Hormone Cure by Sara Gottfried, MD

How Come They're Happy and I'm Not? by Dr. Peter Bongiorno

The Magnesium Miracle by Carolyn Dean, MD, ND

Mastering Leptin by Byron Richards

The Mood Cure by Julia Ross, MA

Practical Paleo by Diane Sanfilippo, BS, NC

Salt, Sugar, Fat by Michael Moss

The Schwarzbein Principle by Dr. Diana Schwarzbein

The 7 Day Detox Miracle by Peter Bennett, MD, and Stephen Barrie, ND

Trust Your Gut by Gregory Plotnikoff, MD, and Dr. Mark Weisberg, PhD

21 Day Sugar Detox by Diane Sanfilippo, BS, NC

The Unhealthy Truth by Robyn O'Brien

The Virgin Diet by JJ Virgin

What Your Doctor May Not Tell You about Heart Disease by Mark C. Houston, MD, MS

Wheat Belly by Dr. William Davis

Why Zebras Don't Get Ulcers by Robert M. Sapolsky

Your Personal Paleo Code by Chris Kresser

Cookbooks

Against All Grain by Danielle Walker

Cultured Food Life by Donna Schwenk

It's All Good by Gwyneth Paltrow (when soy milk is called for, replace with another nondairy option)

Nourishing Traditions by Sally Fallon, with Mary G. Enig, PhD

Quinoa Revolution by Patricia Green and Carolyn Hemming

Super Foods by Lee Holmes

✑ References ✐

Introduction

S. H. Ahmed, K. Guillem, Y. Vandaele, "Sugar Addiction: Pushing the Drug-Sugar Analogy to the Limit." *Curr Opin Clin Nutr Metab Care*, July 2013: 16.

"Artificial Sweeteners May Do More Than Sweeten: It Can Affect How the Body Reacts to Glucose." *ScienceDaily*, 29 May 2013.

D. Chapelot, "The Role of Snacking in Energy Balance: A Biobehavioral Approach." *J Nutr*, January 2011.

S. P. Fowler, et al., "Fueling the Obesity Epidemic? Artificially Sweetened Beverage Use and Long-Term Weight Gain." *Obesity* (Silver Spring, Md.), 2008.

Joseph Mercola, "Artificial Sweeteners May be Worse than Sugar for Diabetics." *Mercola.com*, August 9, 2012.

——— "Aspartame Pathway." *Mercola.com*, February 18, 2013.

U. Ravnskov, "The Questionable Role of Saturated and Polyunsaturated Fatty Acids in Cardiovascular Disease." *J. Clin Epidemiol*, June 1998.

L. M. Redman et al., "Metabolic and Behavioral Compensations in Response to Caloric Restriction: Implications for the Maintenance of Weight Loss." *PLoS ONE, 2009.*

S. D. Stellman, L. Garfinkel, "Artificial Sweetener Use and One Year Weight Change Among Women." *Prev Med*, March 15, 1986.

H. Yang et. al., "Risk Factors for Gallstone Formation During Rapid Loss of Weight." *Digestive Diseases and Sciences*, June 1992.

Qing Yang, "Gain Weight by 'Going Diet?' Artificial Sweeteners and the Neurobiology of Sugar Cravings," *Yale J Biol Med*, June 2010.

Chapter One: Break Up with Sugar

"Added Sugars." American Heart Association.

Daniel Becker, "Suppress Deadly After-Meal Blood Sugar Surges." *Life Extension Magazine*, February 2012.

J. V. Bjornholt, G. Erikssen, E. Aaser et al., "Fasting Blood Glucose: An Underestimated Risk Factor for Cardiovascular Death. Results from a 22-Year Follo-Up of Healthy Nondiabetic Men." *Diabetes Care*, Jan. 22, 1999.

Miller Bock, "NIH Study Shows how Insulin Stimulates Fat Cells to Take in Glucose." *NIH NEWS*, September 7, 2010.

Cristina Carvalho et al., "Increased Susceptibility to Amyloid-β Toxicity in Rat Brain Microvascular Endothelial Cells under Hyperglycemic Conditions." *Journal of Alzheimer's Disease,* October 2013.

Bacon Chow, Howard Stone, "The Relationship of Viatamin B12 to Carbohydrate Metabolism and Diabetes Mellitus." *The American Journal of Clinical Nutrition,* July 1957.

"Chromium." NYU Langone Medical Center, 2011.

R. Crescenzo et al., "Fructose Supplementation Worsens the Deleterious Effects of Short Term High Fat Feeding on Hepatic Steatosis and Lipid Metabolism in Adult Rats." *Exp Physiol,* June 27, 2014.

F. W. Danby, "Nutrition and Aging Skin: Sugar and Glycation." *Clin Dermatol,* July-August 2010.

J. C. de Beer, L. Liebenberg, "Does Cancer Risk Increase with HbA1c, Independent of Diabetes?" *British Journal of Cancer,* April 2014.

"Glycemic Index and Glycemic Load for 100+ Foods." Harvard Health Publications.

S. Hooshmand et al., "Effects of Agave Nectar Versus Sucrose on Weight Gain, Adiposity, Blood Glucose, Insulin, and Lipid Responses in Mice." *J Med Food,* July 10, 2014.

Mark C. Houston, *What Your Doctor May Not Tell You About Heart Disease* (New York: Grand Central, 2012).

Barbara V. Howard, Judith Wylie–Rosett, "Sugar and Cardiovascular Disease, A Statement for Healthcare Professionals from the Committee on Nutrition of the Council on Nutrition, Physical Activity, and Metabolism of the American Heart Association." *Circulation,* 2002.

"Insulin Resistance and Prediabetes." National Diabetes Clearinghouse (NDIC).

Alam Khan, et al., "Cinnamon Improves Glucose and Lipids of People with Type 2 Diabetes." *Diabetes Care Journal,* December 2003.

A Markaki et al., "The Role of Serum Magnesium and Calcium on the Association between Adiponectin Levels and All-Cause Mortality in End-Stage Renal Disease Patients," *PLoS ONE.*

Joseph Mercola, "Artificial Sweeteners—More Dangerous Than You Ever Imagined." *Mercola.com,* October 13, 2009.

——— "Low Magnesium May Play Key Role in Diabetes and Insulin Resistance." *Mercola.com,* May 10, 2014.

Michael Moss, *Salt Sugar Fat: How the Food Giants Hooked Us* (New York: Random House, 2013).

E. Noreen et al., "Effects of Supplemental Fish Oil on Resting Metabolic Rate, Body Composition, and Salivary Cortisol in Healthy Adults." *Journal of the International Society of Sports Nutrition,* 2010.

"Profiling Food Consumption in America." *USDA Agriculture Fact Book.*

Byron Richards, "Magnesium Needed for Healthy Adiponectin Levels." *Wellness Resources,* February 9, 2009.

Ron Rosedale, "Wise Up and Stop Eating Your Muscles for Fuel." *Mercola.com,* July 7, 2005.

Julia Ross, *The Mood Cure, The 8-Step Program to Rebalance Your Body Chemistry and End Food Cravings, Weight Gain, and Mood Swings—Naturally*(New York: Penguin, 2012).

"A Scientific Review: The Role of Chromium in Insulin Resistance." *Diabetes educ.,* 2004.

G. Smith et al., "Dietary Omega-3 Fatty Acid Supplementation Increases the Rate of Muscle Protein Synthesis in Older Adults: A Randomized Controlled Trial." *American Journal of Clinical Nutrition,* 2010.

P. D. Tsitouras et al., "High Omega-3 Fat Intake Improves Insulin Sensitivityand Reduces CRP and IL6, but Does Not Affect Other Endocrine Axes in Healthy Older Adults." *Horm Metab Res.,* March 2008.

J. Wang et al. "Dietary Magnesium Intake Improves Insulin Resistance among Non-Diabetic Individuals with Metabolic Syndrome Participating in a Dietary Trial." *Nutrients,* September 2013.

"Vitamin B-6 Pyroxidine." *The World's Healthiest Foods.*

M. B. Voss, J. E. Lavine, "Dietary Fructose in Nonalcoholic Fatty Liver Disease." *Hepatology,* June 2013.

Quanhe Yang, et al., "Added Sugar Intake and Cardiovascular Diseases Mortality among US Adults." *JAMA Intern Med,* 2014.

Chapter Two: Fix Your Fats!

M. L. Assuncao, "Effects of Dietary Coconut Oil on the Biochemical and Anthropometric Profiles of Women Presenting Abdominal Obesity." *Lipids,* July 2009.

Cherie Calbom, Brian Shilhavy, "How to Help Your Thyroid with Virgin Coconut Oil." *Mercola.com,* November 8, 2003.

Michael Eades, "Framingham Follies." *The Blog of Michael R. Eades, M.D.,* September 2006.

Mary Enig and Sally Fallon, *Eat Fat, Lose Fat* (New York: Penguin, 2005).

——— *Nourishing Traditions, The Cookbook that Challenges Politically Correct Nutrition and the Diet Dictocrats* (Washington, DC: NewTrends, 1999).

Bruce Fife, *Coconut Cures* (Colorado Springs: Piccadilly Books, 2005).

H. Firfer, "Study: 'Bad Fat in Fast Foods Clogs Arteries Faster." *CNN Interactive,* July 11, 1998.

Hibbeln et al., "Omega-3 Fatty Acid Deficiencies in Neurodevelopment, Aggression and Autonomic Dysregulation: Opportunities for Intervention." *Int. Rev Psychiatry,* April 2006.

Mark Houston, *What Your Doctor May Not Tell You About Heart Disease*(New York: Grand Central: 2012).

Lori Lipinski, "TakinFear Out of Eating Fat." *Wise Traditions,,* The West A. Price Foundation, April 30, 2003.

Aseem Malhotra, "Saturated Fat is Not the Major Issue." BMJ, 2013.

Joseph Mercola, "The Cholesterol Myths that May Be Harming Your Health." *Mercola.com*, October 22, 2011.

——— "Two Exciting Alzheimer's Advances: A Novel Detection Test Using Peanut Butter, and a Study Evaluating Coconut Oil." *Mercola.com*, November 7, 2013.

F. Nafar, K.M. Mearow, "Coconut Oil Attenuates the Effects of Amyloid-β on Cortical Neurons in Vitro." *J Alzheimers Dis*, 2014.

"Number (in Millions) of Civilian, Noninstitutionalized Persons With Diagnosed Diabetes, 1980-2011." *Diabetes Public Health Resource*, Centers for Disease Control and Prevention.

L. O'Rourke et al., "Insulin and Leptin Acutely Regulate Cholesterol Ester Metabolism in Macrophages by Novel Signaling Pathways." *Diabetes*, May 2001.

David Perlmutter, *Grain Brain* (New York: Little, Brown, 2013).

U. Ravnskov, "High Cholesterol May Protect against Infections and Atherosclerosis." *QJM*, 2013.

Byron Richards, "Magnesium Needed for Healthy Adiponectin Levels." *Wellness Resources*, February 9, 2009.

U. Riserus et al., "Metabolic Effects of Conjugated Linoleic Acid in Humans: The Swedish Experiment." *The American Journal of Clinical Nutrition*, June 2004.

Diana Schwarzbein, Nancy Deville, *The Schwarzbein Principal* (Deerbeach Field, FL: Health Communications, 1999).

Stephen Sinatra and Jonny Bowden, *The Great Cholesterol Myth* (Minneapolis, Fair Winds Press, 2012).

P. Siri-Tarino et al., "Meta-Analysis of Prospective Cohort Studies Evaluating the Association of Saturated Fat with Cardiovascular Disease." *The American Journal of Clinical Nutrition*, January 13, 2010.

M.P. St-Onge et al., "Medium-Chain Triglycerides Increase Energy Expenditure and Decrease Adiposity in Overweight Men." *Obes Res*, March 2003.

University of California, Los Angeles, "Most Heart Attack Patients' Cholesterol Levels Did Not Indicate Cardiac Risk." *ScienceDaily*, January 13, 2009.

R. West, "Better Memory Functioning Associated with Higher Total and LDL Cholesterol Levels in Very Elderly Subjects without the APOE Allele." *The American Journal of Geriatric Psychiatry*, September 2008.

A. Weiss et al. "Serum Total Cholesterol: A Mortality Predictor in Elderly Hospitalized Patients." *Clinical Nutrition*, May 2012.

A. Yadav, M. A. Katarai, V. Saini, "Role of Leptin and Adiponectin in Insulin Resistance." *Clin Chim Acta*, February 2013.

H. Yang et al., "Risk Factors for Gallstone Formation During Rapid Loss of Weight." *Digestive Diseases and Sciences*, June 1992.

Chapter Three: Heal the Gut

Asociación RUVID, "Effects of Antibiotics on Gut Flora Analyzed." *Science-Daily*, January 9, 2013.

G. Canny, B. McCormick, "Bacteria in the Intestine, Helpful Residents or Enemies from Within?" *Infection and Immunity*, May 12, 2000.

Siri Carpenter, "That Gut Feeling." *American Psychological Association*, September 2012.

"Cleveland Clinic Research Shows Gut Bacteria Byproduct Predicts Heart Attack and Stroke." Cleveland Clinic, April 24, 2013.

"Dietary Approaches to Improve Digestive Disorders." *Life Extension.*

"Digestive Disease Statistics for the United States." National Digestive Diseases Information Clearinghouse, September 2013.

Barry Estabrook, "Antibiotics in Your Food: What's Causing the Rise in Antibiotic-Resistant Bacteria in Our Food Supply." Food and Environment Reporting Network, May 1, 2013.

Bruce Fife, *Coconut Cures* (Colorado Springs: Piccadilly Books, 2005).

Denise Grady, "Bacteria in the Intestines May Help Tip the Bathroom Scale, Studies Show." *The New York Times*, March 27, 2013.

Adam Hadhazy, "Think Twice: How the Gut's 'Second Brain' Influences Mood and Well-Being." *Scientific American*, February 12, 2010.

A. R. Lomax, P. C. Calder, "Probiotics, Immune Function, Infection and Inflammation: A Review of the Evidence from Studies Conducted in Humans." *Curr Parm Des.*, 2009.

Howard Markel, "The Real Story Behind Penicillin." *PBS NewsHour*, September 27, 2013.

Oregon State University, "Gut Microbes Closely Linked to Proper Immune Function, Other Health Issues." *ScienceDaily*, September 16, 2013.

Byron Richards, "How Digestive Problems Prevent Weight Loss—The Leptin Diet Weight Loss Challenge #2." April 9, 2012.

——— *Mastering Leptin, Your Guide to Permanent Weight Loss and Optimum Health* (Minneapolis: Wellness Resource Books, 2009).

Rajiv Saini, Santosh Saini, Sugandha Sharma, "Potential of Probiotics in Controlling Cardiovascular Diseases." *J Cardiovasc Dis Res*, October–December 2010.

S. A. Walter et al., "Abdominal Pain Is Associated with Anxiety and Depression Scores in a Sample of the General Adult Population with No Signs of Organic Gastrointestinal Disease." *Neurogastroenterol Motil.*, September 2013.

W. H. Wilson Tang et al. "Intestinal Microbial Metabolism of Phosphatidylcholine and Cardiovascular Risk." *New England Journal of Medicine*, 2013.

Chapter Four: Identify Food Intolerances

Jonathan Brostoff, Linda Gamlin, *Food Allergies and Food Intolerance* (Rochester, VT: Healing Arts Press, 2000).

Lester Crawford, "Understanding Biotechnology in Agriculture." *Economic Perspectives*, 2003.

D'Aloisio et al., "Soy Formula Associated with Higher Risk of Fibroids in Women." *Environmental Health News*, February 1, 2010.

F. W. Danby, "Acne, Dairy and Cancer: The 5alpha-P Link." *Dermatoendocrinol*, January 2009.

William Davis, *Wheat Belly* (New York: Rodale, 2014).

Dinesh K Dhanwal et al., "Epidemiology of Hip Fracture: Worldwide Geographic Variation." *Indian Journal of Orthopaedics*, Jan-Mar 2011.

D. Feskanich, W. C. Willett, M. J. Stampfer, G. A. Colditz, "Milk Dietary Calcium, and Bone Fractures in Women, a 12Year Study." *American Journal of Public Health*, 1997.

"Genetically Engineered Foods, a Statement of James H. Maryanski, PhD before the Subcommittee on Basic Research, House Committee on Science." U.S. Food and Drug Administration, October 19, 1999.

Gilles-Eric Seralini, "RETRACTED: Long Term Toxicity of a Roundup Herbicide and a Roundup-Tolerant Genetically Modified Maize." *Food and Chemical Toxicology*, November 2012.

"GMO Facts," and "What is GMO" The Non GMO Project.

Mark Hyman, "Gluten: What You Don't Know Might Kill You." *DrHyman.com*, February 15, 2013.

I. Jakobsson, "Unusual Presentation of Adverse Reactions to Cow's Milk Proteins." *Klin Padiatr.*, July 1985.

Lindsey Konkel, "Could Eating Too Much Soy be Bad for You?" *Scientific American*, November 2003.

Chris Kresser, "The Thyroid-Gut Connection." *ChrisKresser.com*.

Amy Joy Lanou, "Should Dairy Be Recommended as Part of a Healthy Vegetarian Diet? Counterpoint." *Am J Clin Nutr.*, May 2009.

Loyola University Health System, "Spring Allergies Linked to Specific Food Allergies, Says Specialist." *ScienceDaily*, April 7, 2014.

Joseph Mercola, "The Critical Role of Wheat in Human Disease." *Mercola.com*, January 16, 2010.

——— "The Health Dangers of Soy." *The Huffpost Healthy Living*, August 23, 2012.

Tom O' Bryan, "The Gluten-Thyroid Connection." *The Thyroid Sessions, The Second Opinion Series*.

David Perlmutter, *Grain Brain* (New York: Little, Brown, 2013).

A. Pusztai et al., "Antinutritive Effects of Wheat-Germ Agglutinin and Other N-acetylglucosamine-Specific Lectin." *Br. J Nutrition*, July 1993.

Jessica Rubino, "7 Gluten Free Statistics You Need to Know." *NewHope360*, May 20, 2013.

Mary Shomon, "All About Goitrogens,m Why Thyroid Patients Are Warned About Cruciferous Vegetables." *About.com Thyroid Disease*, June 2, 2014.

Chapter Five: Lose the Toxic Weight

J. Bunyan, E. A. Murrell, P. P. Shah, "The Induction of Obesity in Rodents by Means of Monosodium Glutamate." *Br J Nutr*, January 1976.

Radan Bruha, Karel Dvorak, Jaromir Petrtyl, "Alcoholic Liver Disease." *World J Hepatol*, Mar 27, 2012.

"Fatty Liver Disease." *WebMD*.

Max Goldberg, "Another Reason to Eat Organic—Decrease Pesticide Exposure by 90%." The Cornucopia Institute, May 19, 2014.

Jane Higdon, "Lipoic Acid." Linus Pauling Institute, April 2006.

Wendee Holtcamp, "Obesogens: An Environmental Link to Obesity." *Environmental Health Perspectives*, February 2002.

"Non Alcoholic Fatty Liver Disease." American Liver Foundation, October 4, 2011.

Norwegian School of Veterinary Science, "Environmental Toxins Affect the Body's Hormone Systems." *Science Daily*, July 6, 2010.

Olney, "Brain Lesions, Obesity, and Other Disturbances in Mice Treated with Monosodium Glutamate." *Science*, May 1969.

"Environmental, Energetic, and Economic Comparisons of Organic and Conventional Farming Systems." *BioScience*, 2005.

D. Pimentel, M. Pimentel, *Food, Energy, and Society*, 3rd ed. (Boca Raton, FL: CRC Press, 2008).

Byron Richards, "Why Toxins and Waste Products Impede Weight Loss—The Leptin Weight Loss Challenge #3." *Wellness Resources*, April 16, 2012.

R. A. Rudel et al., "Food Packaging and Bisphenol A and Bis(2-Ethylhexyl) Phthalate Exposure: Findings from a Dietary Intervention." *Environmental Health Perspectives*, July 1, 2011.

"Superbugs Invade American Supermarkets." *Guide to Climate Change and Health*, Environmental Working Group, 2013.

Bryan Walsh, "The Perils of Plastic." *Time*, April 1, 2010.

Chapter Six: Put Out the Fire of Inflammation

Rachel Champeau, "Most Heart Attack Patients' Cholesterol Levels Did Not Indicate Cardiac Risk." *UCLA Newsroom*, January 12, 2009.

Floyd Chilton, *Win the War Within* (New York: Rodale, 2006).

Christine Gorman, Alice Park, Kristina Dell, "Health: The Fires Within." *Time*, February 23, 2004.

Mark Houston, *What Your Doctor May Not Tell You About Heart Disease* (New York: Grand Central, 2012).

Mark Hyman, "Inflammation: How to Cool the Fire Inside of You That's Making You Fat and Diseased." *MarkHyman.com*, January 27, 2012.

Peter Libby, Paul M. Ridker, Attilio Maseri, "Inflammation and Atherosclerosis." *Circulation*, 2002.

"The New Science behind America's Deadliest Diseases." *Wall Street Journal*, July 16, 2012.

Ohio State University, "Omega-3 Supplements May Slow a Biological Effect of Aging." *Science Daily*, October 1, 2012.

David Perlmutter, *Grain Brain* (New York: Little, Brown, 2013).

E. Selvin, N. P. Paynter, T. P. Erlinger, "The Effect of Weight Loss on C-Reactive Protein: A Systematic Review." *The Archives of Internal Medicine*, "January 8, 2007."

Chapter Seven: Stop the Madness

O. M. Buxton et al., "Adverse Metabolic Consequences in Humans of Prolonged Sleep Restriction Combined with Circadian Disruption." *Science Translational Medicine*, 2012.

Wayne Dyer, "Stress Begone!" *Drwaynedyer.com/blog*, June 25, 2010.

"Facts About Insomnia." The National Sleep Foundation.

Peter J. Gianaros et al., "An Inflammatory Pathway Links Atherosclerotic Cardiovascular Disease Risk to Neural Activity Evoked by the Cognitive Regulation of Emotion." *Biological Psychiatry*, May 1, 2014.

Carolyn Gregoire, "The Daily Habit of These Outrageously Successful People." *Huffington Post*, July 5, 2013.

Tsonwin Hai et al., "Transcription Factor ATF3 Links Host Adaptive Response to Breast Cancer Metastasis." *J Clin Invest*, 2013.

Hyo Jung Kang et al., "Decreased Expression of Synapse-Related Genes and Loss of Synapses in Major Depressive Disorder." *Nature Medicine*, 2012.

P. Lee et al., "Temperature-Acclimated Brown Adipose Tissue Modulates Insulin Sensitivity in Humans." *Diabetes*, June 2014.

Howard LeWine, "Alcohol: A Heart Disease-Cancer Balancing Act." *Harvard Health Publications*, Feb 15, 2013.

Nicholas Perricone, "Cortisol, the Death Hormone," *Daily Perricone*, March 12, 2012.

G. Sigthorsson et al., "Intestinal Permeability and Inflammation in Patients on NSAIDS." *Gut*, Oct. 1998.

Sharad Taheri et al., "Short Sleep Duration is Associated with Reduced Leptin, Elevated Ghrelin, and Increased Body Mass Index." *PLoS Med*, December 2004.

Lawrence Wilson, "Physical Tests Associated with Adrenal Gland Activity." The Center for Development, November 2013.

"Workplace Stress." The American Institute of Stress, *Stress.org/workplace-stress*.

Chapter Eight: Ditch the Convenience Foods

Peter Brøndum-Jacobsen, et al., "25 Hodroxyvitamin D Levels and Risk of Ischemic Heart Disease, Myocardial Infarction, and Early Death." Teriosclerosis, Thrombosis, and Vascular Biology, August 30, 2012.

C. Garland, et al., "Vitamin D for Cancer Prevention: Global Perspective." Annals of Epidemiology, August 2014.

Elson Haas, Staying Healthy with Nutrition (Berkeley, CA: Celestial Arts, 2006).

H. C. Hung et al., "Fruit and Vegetable Intake and Risk of Major Chronic Disease." J Natl Cancer Inst, 2004.

L. Noguerira et al., "Epicatechin Enhances Fatigue Resistance and Oxidative Capacity in Mouse Muscle." The Journal of Physiology, July 25, 2011.

Oyinlola Oyebode et al., "Fruit and Vegetable Consumption and All-Cause, Cancer and CVD Mortality: Analysis of Health Survey for England Data." J Epidemiol Community Health, March 31, 2014.

University College London, "New Evidence Linking Fruit and Vegetable Consumption with Lower Mortality." ScienceDaily, March 31, 2014.

"Vegetables and Fruits: Get Plenty Every Day." Harvard School of Public Health.

Marianne C. Verhaar et al., "5-Methyltetrahydrofolate, The Active Form of Folic Acid, Restores Endothelial Function in Familial Hypercholesterolemia." Circulation, 1998.

David Weigle et al., "A High-Protein Diet Induces Sustained Reductions in Appetite, ad libitum Caloric Intake, and Body Weight Despite Compensatory Changes in Diurnal Plasma Leptin and Ghrelin Concentrations." American Journal of Clinical Nutrition, July 2005.

A. H. Wu et al., "Green Tea and Risk of Breast Cancer in Asian Americans." Int J Cancer, September 10, 2003.

Chapter Nine: Hydrate, Hydrate, Hydrate

Peter Agre, "The Aquaporin Water Channels." Proceedings of the American Thoracic Society, March 2006.

Emily Arnold and Janet Larson, "Bottled Water: Pouring Resources Down the Drain." Earth Policy Institute, February 2, 2006.

"Avoiding Dehydration, Proper Hydration." Cleveland Clinic.

F. Batmanghelidj, Your Body's Many Cries for Water (Decatur, GA: Global Health Solutions, 2008).

"Bottled Water Pricey in More Ways than One." Worldwatch Institute, July 13, 2014.

"Drinking Water Contaminants." United States Environmental Protection Agency.

"Endocrine Disruptors." National Institute of Environmental Health Sciences.

A. B. Goodman, et al., "Behaviors and Attitudes Associated with Low Drinking Water Intake Among US Adults, Food Attitudes and Behaviors Survey, 2007." Preventing Chronic Disease, 2013.

"Is Eight Enough? U Researcher Says Drink Up and Tells Why." University of Utah Health Care, Jan 14, 2003.

B. Popkin, K. D'Anci, and I. Rosenberg, "Water, Hydration and Health." *Nutr. Rev.*, August 2010.

James Stockand, "Vasopressin Regulation of Renal Sodium Extretion." *Kidney Int.*, 2010.

Chapter Ten: Exercise Smarter (Not Harder)

John A Babraj et al., "Extremely Short Duration High Intensity Interval Training Substantially Improves Insulin Action in Young Healthy Males." *BMC Endocr Disord.*, 2009.

A. J. Bidwell et al., "Physical Activity Offsets the Negative Effects of a High Fructose Diet." *Med Sci Sports Exerc*, May 2014.

Framson et al., "Development and Validation of the Mindful Eating Questionnaire." *Journal of the American Dietetic Association*, 2009.

Hamilton, Hamilton, and Zderic, "Role of Low Energy Expenditure and Sitting in Obesity, Metabolic Syndrome, Type 2 Diabetes, and Cardiovascular Disease." *Diabetes*, 2007.

Robert M. Sapolsky, *Why Zebras Don't Get Ulcers* (New York: Henry Holt and Company, 2004).

James Vlahos, "Is Sitting a Lethal Activity?" *The New York Times Magazine*, April 14, 2011.

Chapter 11: Metabolism Hacks

F. Bellise, R. McDevitt, A. M. Prentice, "Meal Frequency and Energy Balance." *Br. J Nutr*, April 1997.

Megumi Hatori et al., "Time Restricted Feeding without Reducing Caloric Intake Prevents Metabolic Diseases in Mice Fed a High Fat Diet." *Cell Metabolism*, May 17, 2012.

Byron J. Richards, *Mastering Leptin* (Minneapolis: Wellness Resource Books, 2009).

"Salk Study May Offer Drug-Free Intervention to Prevent Obesity and Diabetes." Salk Institute for Biological Studies, May 17, 2012.

Alice G. Walton, "Why is Skipping Breakfast So Bad for Our Heart Health?" *Forbes*, July 23, 2013.

❦ About the Author ❧

Sara Vance is a certified nutritionist and the founder of the company Rebalance Life LLC. She is a regular contributor to Fox News Health, San Diego, as well as MindBodyGreen and eHow. She has worked in collaboration with doctors, taught at schools and community centers, created videos for Gaiam TV, and sees individual clients. Visit her at *www.rebalancelife.com.*

❧ To Our Readers ❧

Conari Press, an imprint of Red Wheel/Weiser, publishes books on topics ranging from spirituality, personal growth, and relationships to women's issues, parenting, and social issues. Our mission is to publish quality books that will make a difference in people's lives—how we feel about ourselves and how we relate to one another. We value integrity, compassion, and receptivity, both in the books we publish and in the way we do business.

Our readers are our most important resource, and we appreciate your input, suggestions, and ideas about what you would like to see published.

Visit our website at *www.redwheelweiser.com* to learn about our upcoming books and free downloads, and be sure to go to *www.redwheelweiser.com/newsletter* to sign up for newsletters and exclusive offers.

You can also contact us at *info@rwwbooks.com*.

Conari Press
an imprint of Red Wheel/Weiser, LLC
665 Third Street, Suite 400
San Francisco, CA 94107